ADVANCED GREEN SMOOTHIES

Better Health Through Unusual Ingredients

A collection of 50 green smoothies using unique superfoods from around the world, for those trying to achieve improved health, increased energy and a stronger immune system.

Duc Vuong, M.D.

 Published by HappyStance Publishing.

Print ISBN-13: 978-0692145388

Print ISBN-10: 0692145389

Contents

Introduction

Why Add Green Smoothies to Your Diet?

A healthy life begins, every single day, with the right breakfast. For much of my career helping people lose weight, I have encouraged one consistent practice: waking up each morning with a tasty green smoothie.

Food trends come and go—what stays consistent is the benefits of whole, natural foods in our diet. Below, I've provided you with 50 unique combinations for smoothies, elixirs and even puddings that can be made within minutes. Each contains ingredients which will help you to fight off disease and live a longer, more active life.

Here are some reasons why you should switch to green smoothies today:

- Green smoothies are loaded with antioxidants, vitamins and minerals.
- Daily fruit and vegetable intake is drastically increased.
- Every green smoothie hydrates and and promotes bowel regularity thanks to plenty of fiber.
- Smoothie prep and cleanup are quick and easy.
- You'll also be motivated to use these fruits, vegetables, and superfoods in the rest of your daily meals.
- From toddlers to octogenarians, green smoothies are great for people of all ages, so preparing them daily can become a family affair.
- Each of the 50 recipes below can be modified to individual tastes.

I intentionally wrote this book without including the macronutrient content like calories, carbohydrates and protein counts. Why? I want you to focus on the nutritional value of the foods you consume, instead of judging them by only a few established conventions. The value of whole foods is so much more than just a few metrics. Make trying the advanced ingredients the goal, not scrutiny of carb content. Make daily smoothie consumption the objective, not food weighing. Turn learning about the unusual ingredients into a passion, as opposed to calorie-counting. This book is meant to be liberating, not limiting.

Superfoods to the Rescue

These 50 green smoothie recipes are designed to do 3 things:

- Make you healthier.
- Ignite your palate.
- Simplify your life.

With this book, I've taken care of one of your meals because a green smoothie can be a complete meal for you. I've introduced many delicious superfoods in the recipes below. Here are a few highlights:

Acai

The acai (ah-sigh-EE) berry comes to us from the rainforests of South America. These berries became a commercial sensation when they were first featured on Oprah. Like any other berry, they are packed with antioxidants and fiber. In comparison to a regular berry like blueberries, acai contain 3 times the antioxidant levels. Those powerful plant compounds are also connected to anti-aging benefits and lowering of cholesterol. Both powdered acai and smoothie packs are available at most grocery stores.

Bee Pollen

The foods created by bees are some of Earth's true wonders. Bee pollen is a combination of the pollen collected by the bees from flowers, and a small dose of the nectar secreted by their salivary glands. It contains more protein than any animal source. It provides amazing natural allergy relief and is antifungal and antibacterial.

Chlorella

This blue-green algae superfood is rich with phytonutrients, including amino acids, chlorophyll, beta-carotene, potassium, phosphorous, biotin, magnesium and the B-complex vitamins. Chlorella benefits the entire body by supporting healthy hormone function, helping to negate the effects of chemotherapy and radiation, lowering blood pressure and cholesterol, and aiding in the detoxification of our bodies.

Dandelion Greens

Aren't dandelion greens weeds? Not at all. If you haven't tried them before, you're going to fall in love with their earthy, slightly bitter taste. Like other greens, they are low in calories and high in fiber. They sport high levels of vitamin C, vitamin K and vitamin A. They are great in smoothies, and if you have more to spare, make yourself a cup of highly nutritious dandelion tea.

Goji Berry

Also called the wolfberry, goji is a bright orange-red berry that comes from a shrub that is native to China. In Asia, goji berries have been eaten for generations in the hope of living longer. Low in calories, fat-free, a good source of fiber and antioxidants, goji berry benefits include the ability to help fight disease, manage your weight, treat diabetes, and experience better digestion.

Hemp Hearts

What are hemp hearts? They are the fully edible insides of hemp seeds, and they also contain a lot of protein. They're packed with essential fatty acids, and soluble and insoluble fiber. The calories, complex carbs and protein in hemp hearts turn them into tiny energy blasters. Eat them to curb hunger and feel invigorated all day long.

Lucuma

Lucuma powder comes from the lucuma fruit, native to Peru, Ecuador, and Chile. In addition to serving as a natural sweetener, it provides 14 essential trace elements. If you are diabetic, lucuma will not raise blood sugar levels.

Maca Powder

Maca is a plant native to Peru. It is shaped like a turnip or radish but is more closely related to broccoli and cauliflower. Maca is a relatively new superfood on the market, but most health food stores sell it in powdered or liquid form. It is highly nutritious, containing lots of vitamin C (133% of the RDI), copper, iron, and potassium. It is low in fat but high in fiber, protein and carbohydrates.

Matcha Tea

Matcha powder likely rings a bell as a now-popular alternative to coffee, but there is so much more to this glowing green substance. Young leaves are plucked from shade-grown Camellia sinensis plants, then steamed, rolled, and deveined before being ground into powder. Being super high in antioxidants, this magical powder could possibly help prevent cancer, promote weight loss, improve exercise performance, lower blood pressure, and detoxify the body. Amino acid L-theanine provides alertness without the jitters of caffeine.

Medjool Dates

Packed full of vitamins, minerals and fiber, the health benefits of medjool dates are remarkable. These edible sweet fruits of the date palm tree make great natural sweeteners and sugar alternatives, but they're not just delicious. Potassium, iron, and magnesium, help lower cholesterol and boost energy.

Moringa

Moringa is a plant that is native to the sub-Himalayan areas of India and Bangladesh. It is also grown in the tropics. The leaves, bark, flowers, fruit, seeds, and root are used to make medicine. It is used for arthritis, asthma, constipation, diabetes, stomach ulcers, and a host of other ailments. It can also be applied topically to treat abscesses, athlete's foot, dandruff, warts, and wounds.

Spirulina

This blue-green algae is a freshwater plant that is now one of the most researched, and most talked about superfoods today. Spirulina is renowned for its intense flavor and even more powerful nutrition profile. It helps detoxify heavy metals, especially arsenic, promotes weight loss, improves blood pressure, and gives an amazing energy boost.

Tahini

Tahini is a Middle Eastern paste made from ground sesame seeds. It is incredibly versatile, lending its nutty richness to everything from salad dressings to cookies.

Tofu

Tofu comes from soybeans and is a great source of non-animal protein. It is also great for smoothies because it is flavorless. Use the soft texture for better blending.

Wheatgrass

This powerful plant turns into a living emerald liquid or potent powder. I can't say enough about what makes wheatgrass so special. It contains numerous essential minerals known to man. The juice is up to 70% chlorophyll, a blood builder with potential to slow the aging process. It contains a whopping 17 amino acids, and therefore is a mainstay of many body builders worldwide.

Recipe Prep Tips

- Use an emulsifying blender, like a NutriBullet or NutriNinja. A high-end blender might also have a smoothie function.
- Chop thicker ingredients before blending.
- Use fresh and raw ingredients whenever possible.
- If fresh ingredients are not available, frozen is the next best option.
- If frozen fruit is used, then you do not need to use ice cubes.
- Add honey or dates if more sweetness is desired. Avoid artificial sweeteners, including Stevia.
- Adjust the amount of liquid base for desired thickness.
- You can substitute any leafy green for your favorite. For example, if you don't like kale, then you might try arugula instead.
- You can add or switch any of the powder ingredients.
- If you are using a protein powder, be careful because the powder might add an undesirable taste.
- Use unflavored supplements and powders whenever possible.
- You may substitute any liquid base that is in the recipe, to achieve endless combinations.

Introducing smoothies to your daily diet will invigorate and inspire you. There simply is no better way to get all your vitamins, minerals, and fiber delivered quickly and naturally. As a surgeon who sees many of his patients struggling to lose weight, I recommend them to everyone preoperatively with amazing results. If the smoothies help my morbidly obese patients, I know they can help you. I even give them to my children in the mornings instead of a “typical” breakfast.

A daily smoothie leads to other good habits, like keeping a pantry and a fridge full of fresh produce. Your family will quickly get on board with this new healthy lifestyle. A daily smoothie is an affordable investment in good health, and it will pay in dividends throughout your life.

THE SMOOTHIES…

1. Chocolate Matcha Smoothie

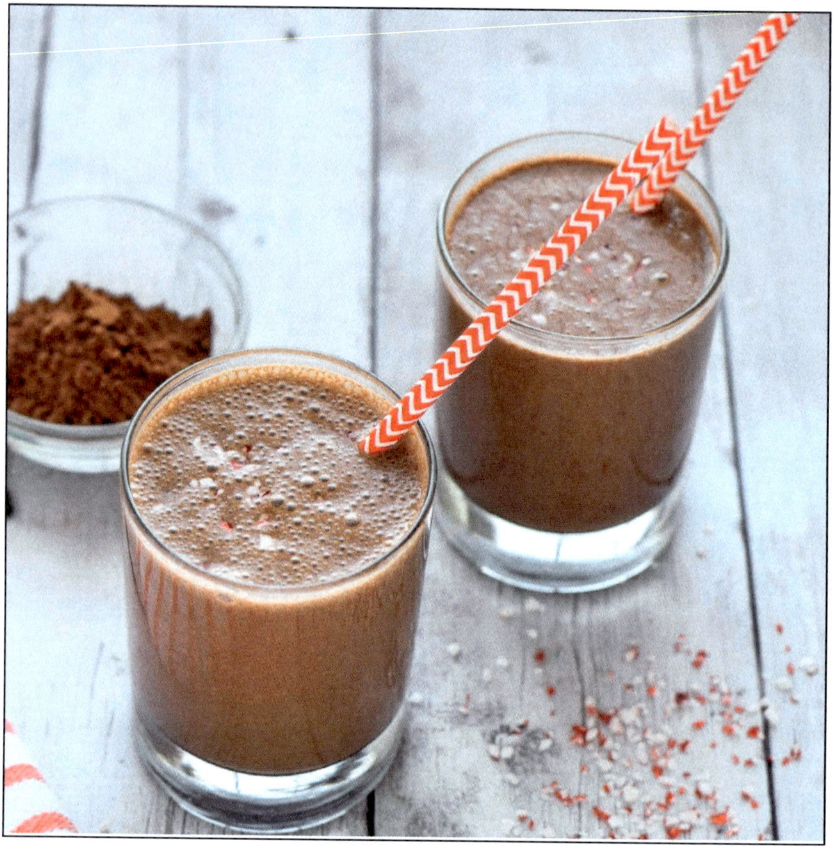

We will start off easy. This smoothie is both a filling meal replacement, and an efficient energy booster with the added Matcha powder. It tastes like a healthy chocolate milkshake – the greens disappear right into the mix, and don't affect its creamy goodness.

Ingredients

- 2 cups spinach, loosely packed
- 1 cup blueberries, fresh or frozen
- 1 tablespoon unsweetened cocoa powder
- ½ cup unsweetened almond milk
- ½ cup ice
- 1 tsp raw honey
- 1 tbsp. Matcha powder (use high-quality premium or café-grade Matcha for smoothies)

Your Notes

2. Tofu Flaxseed Almond Butter Smoothie

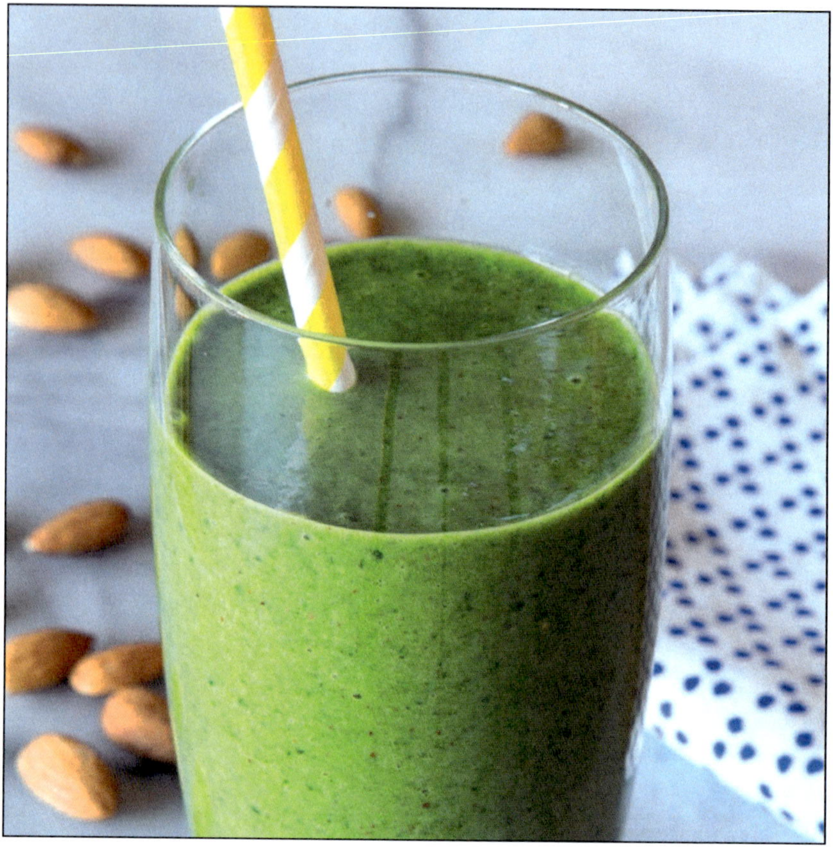

If you've never tried soft tofu in a smoothie, I highly recommend it. It is so neutral in flavor that the taste of the fruit and almond butter shines through instead. It also offers a nice protein boost!

Ingredients

- ½ cup soft tofu
- 2 tablespoons natural almond butter
- 2 cups spinach, loosely packed
- 1 banana
- 3 strawberries
- 1/2 cup ice
- 1 tsp ground flaxseed

Your Notes

3. Acai Coconut Smoothie

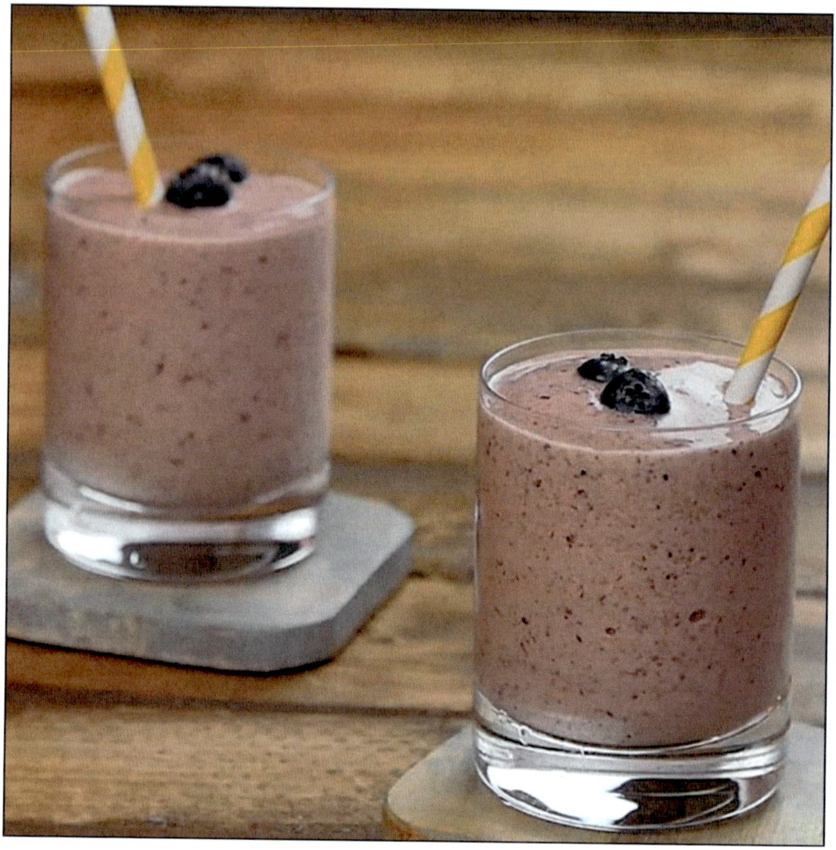

Hemp protein powder and acai powder can both be found in health food stores, and online. The ground flaxseed and coconut milk deliver essential fatty acids, making this smoothie a perfect marriage of protein, carbs and healthy fats.

Ingredients

- ½ cup blueberries
- 2-3 strawberries
- ¼ cup coconut milk
- 1 cup kale with ribs removed
- 1 tbsp. hemp protein powder
- 1 tbsp. ground flaxseed
- 2 tbsp. chia seeds
- 1.5 tsp cinnamon
- 1.5 tbsp. acai powder
- 1 banana
- ½ cup ice

Your Notes

4. Super Green Smoothie

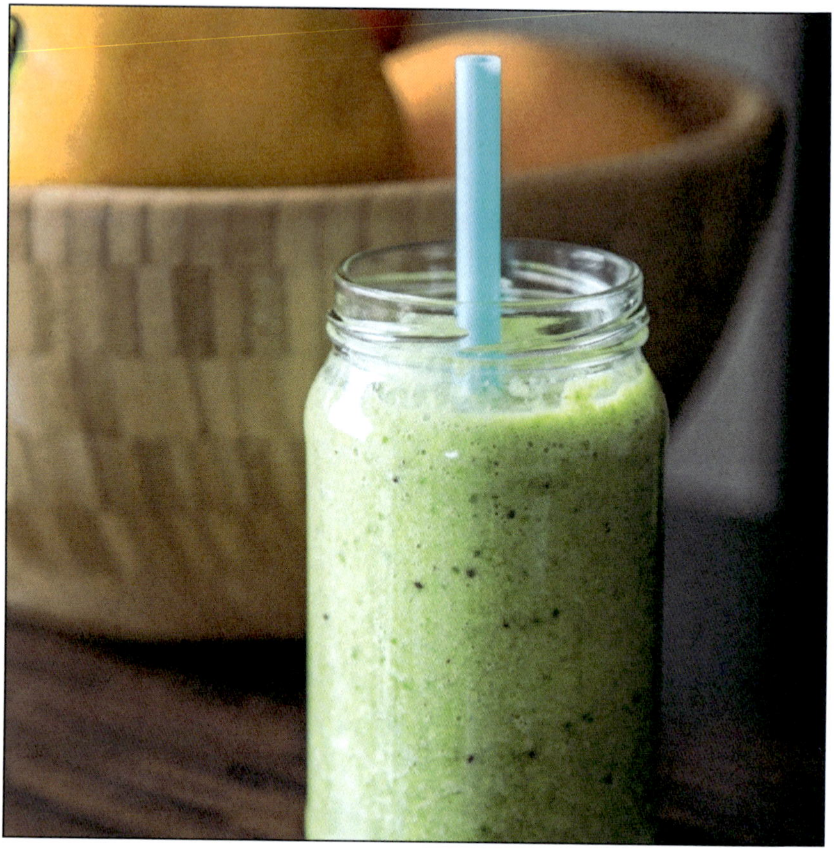

This smoothie is an unbeatable powerhouse, and a great way to start your day. Maca is a cruciferous vegetable native to the Andes in Peru. When ground into powder, it can act as an adaptogen, delivering micronutrients and high levels of antioxidants. Together with the wheatgrass powder, this superfood smoothie delivers a blast of good health.

Ingredients

- 1 cup almond milk
- 1 banana
- 2 cups spinach
- 1 kiwi
- 1 tbsp. chia seeds
- 1 tsp maca powder
- 1 tbsp. wheatgrass powder
- ½ cup ice

Your Notes

5. Vanilla Green Valley Shake

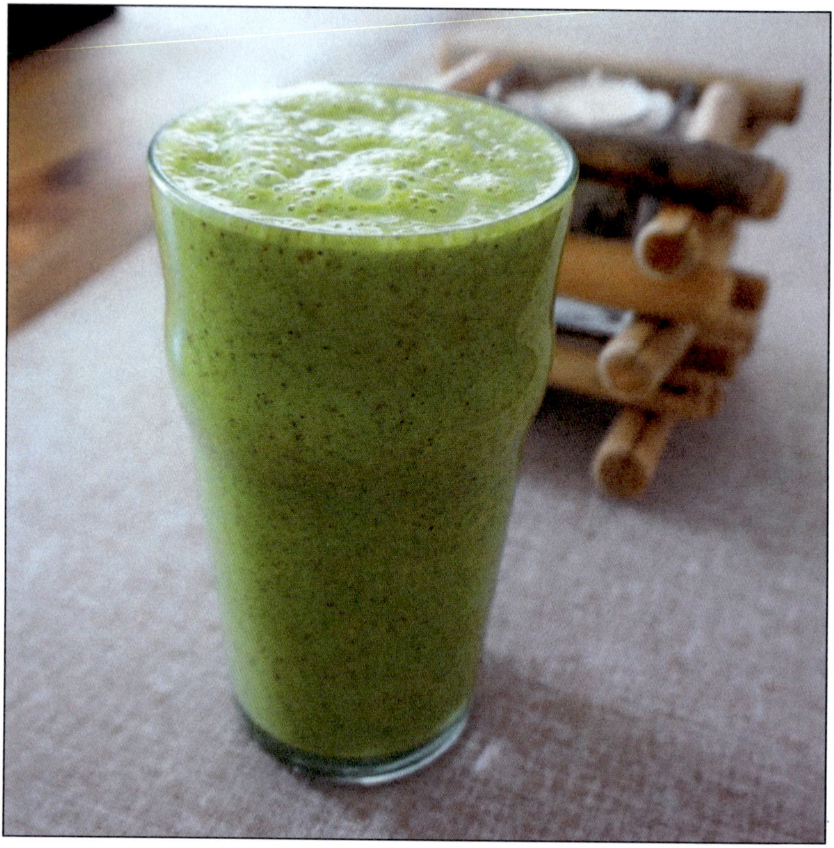

This vibrant green smoothie is fueled with the benefits of soy protein powder, which is a plant protein source. Spinach loads you up with iron, and almond butter delivers healthy fats and a nutty twist to this tasty smoothie.

Ingredients

- 1 cup vanilla almond milk
- 1.5 tbsp. almond butter
- 1 scoop soy vanilla protein powder
- 1 banana
- 1.5 cups spinach
- 1 cup ice

Your Notes

6. Citrus Kale Smoothie

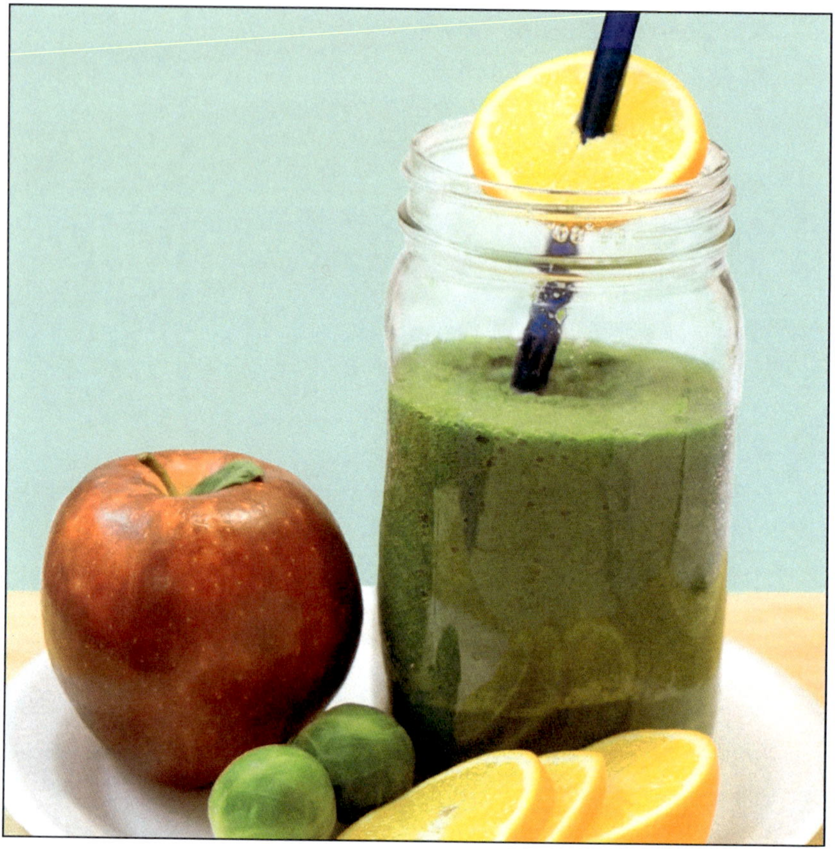

The grapefruit, apples, and mango give a sweet-tart kick that masks the kale. Hemp hearts and coconut oil yield the ideal omega-3 and omega-6 fatty acid balance your brain requires for good functioning.

Ingredients

- ¼ cup red grapefruit juice
- 1 apple, seeded and quartered
- 1.5 cups kale, ribs removed
- 1 celery stalk, chopped
- 1 cup cucumber, diced
- ½ cup mango
- 4 tbsp. hemp hearts
- ¼ cup mint leaves
- 4 ice cubes
- ½ tbsp. coconut oil

Your Notes

7. Tropical Power Smoothie

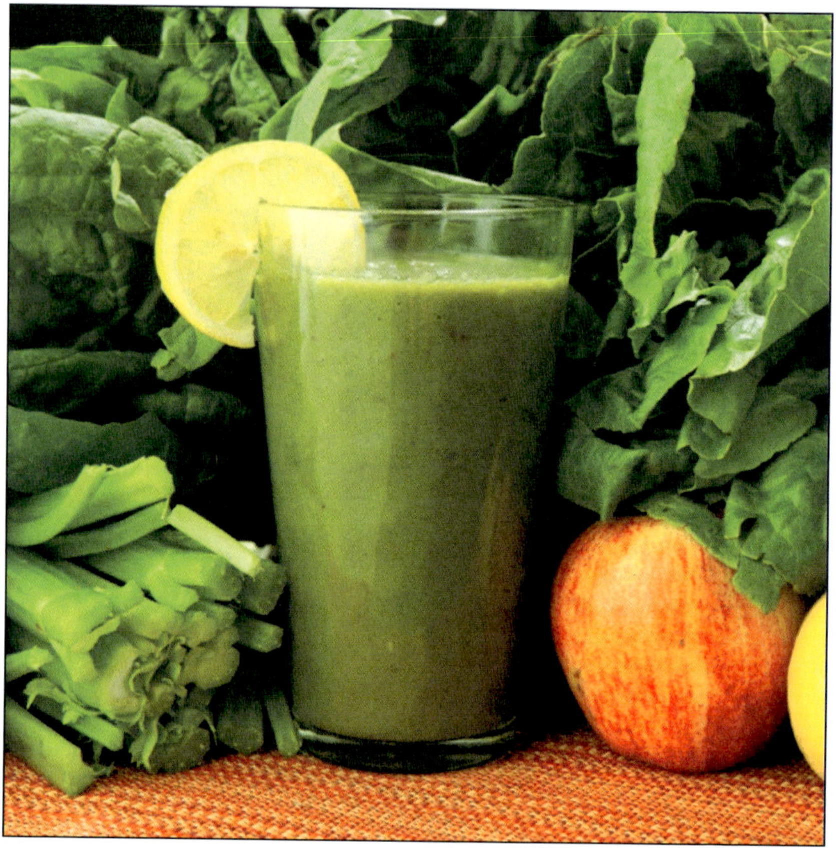

This vibrant kale AND spinach smoothie is essential for a nutrient-packed, protein-powered morning. Chia seeds promote a healthy balance of omega-3 fatty acids and omega-6 fatty acids.

Ingredients

- 2 cups spinach
- 1 ¼ cup vanilla almond milk
- 1 cup kale
- 1 cup diced pineapple
- ½ tbsp. chia seeds
- 1 scoop soy protein powder
- ½ cup ice

Your Notes

8. Kiwi Ginger Green Smoothie

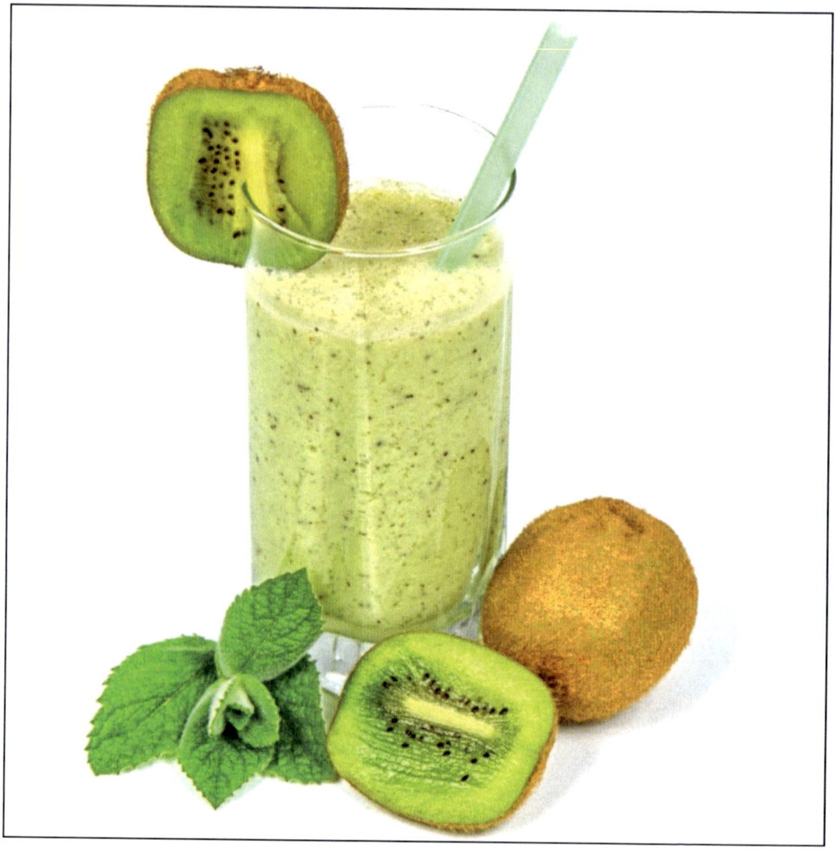

Most of us buy our ginger powdered or processed in some other form, but I highly encourage you to make fresh ginger a part of your daily routine. It can ease joint and muscle pain, regulate blood sugar and even help to lower your cholesterol. Combined here with apple and kiwi, it will leave you tingling.

Ingredients

- 2 kiwis, peeled
- 1 apple, seeded and quartered
- 2 cups kale, ribs removed
- ½ cup cilantro
- 1 large slice fresh ginger, peeled
- 1 cup almond milk
- ½ cup ice

Your Notes

9. Apple Sour Smoothie with Chlorella

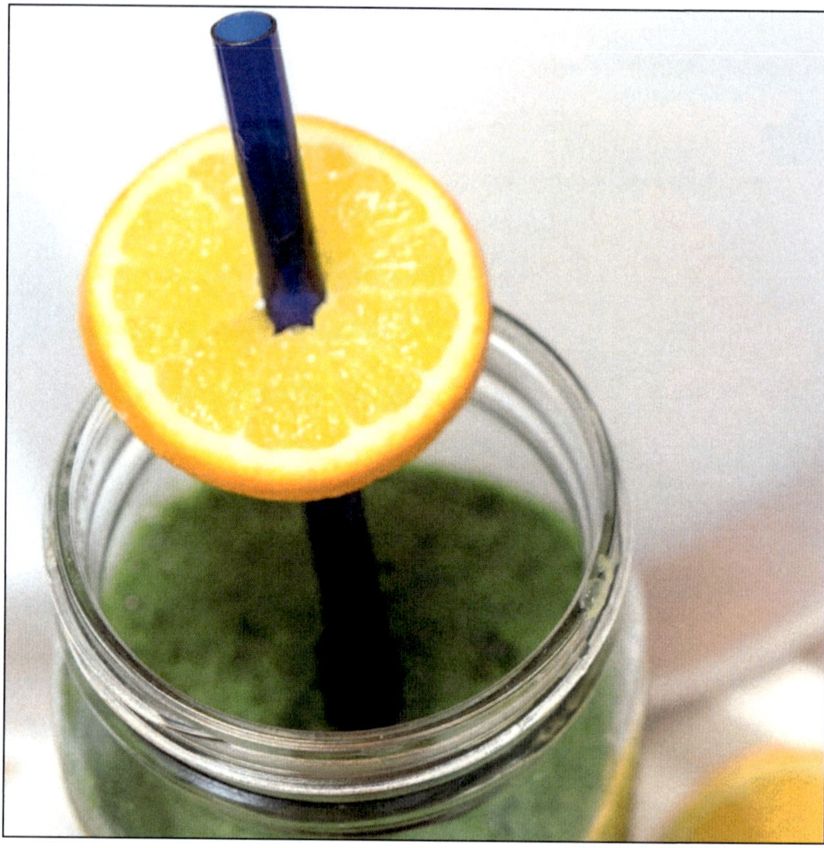

Chlorella is a superfood, derived from rich freshwater algae. It aids the body in the detoxification process, promotes heart health, supports normal hormonal function, and so much more. You will love this fresh lemony combination for sipping as the sun rises.

Ingredients

- 1 cup lettuce (mixed greens are recommended, or spinach works as well)
- 2 apples, seeded and quartered
- 2 kiwis
- 1/4 lemon, including peel & rind
- 1 tbsp. chlorella
- 1 cup ice

Your Notes

10. Flax Kiwi Spinach Smoothie

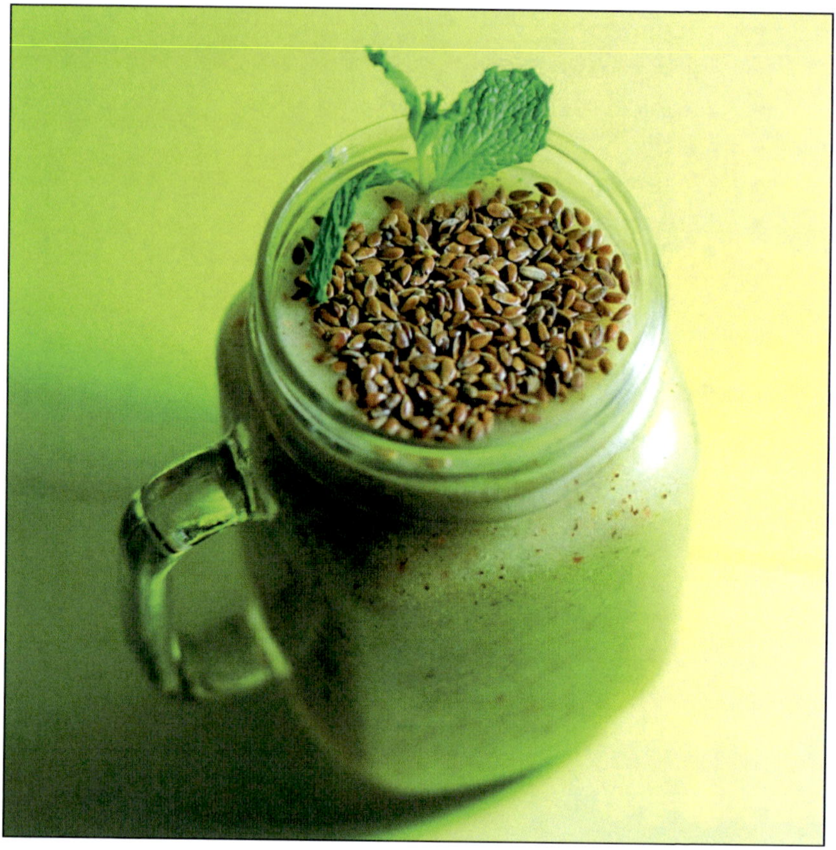

Every tablespoon of ground flaxseed packs about 1.8 grams of plant omega-3's, also known as heart-healthy fats. It also sports high fiber and lignin levels. Preliminary studies link it to possible advances in the fight against heart disease, diabetes and breast cancer. When ground, that makes this tiny seed one of the most powerful dietary additives on the market.

Ingredients

- 1 cup spinach
- 1 apple, seeded and quartered
- 1 banana
- 1 stalk celery
- 3 kiwis
- 3 tbsp. ground flaxseed
- 1 cup ice

Your Notes

11. Parsley Apple Smoothie

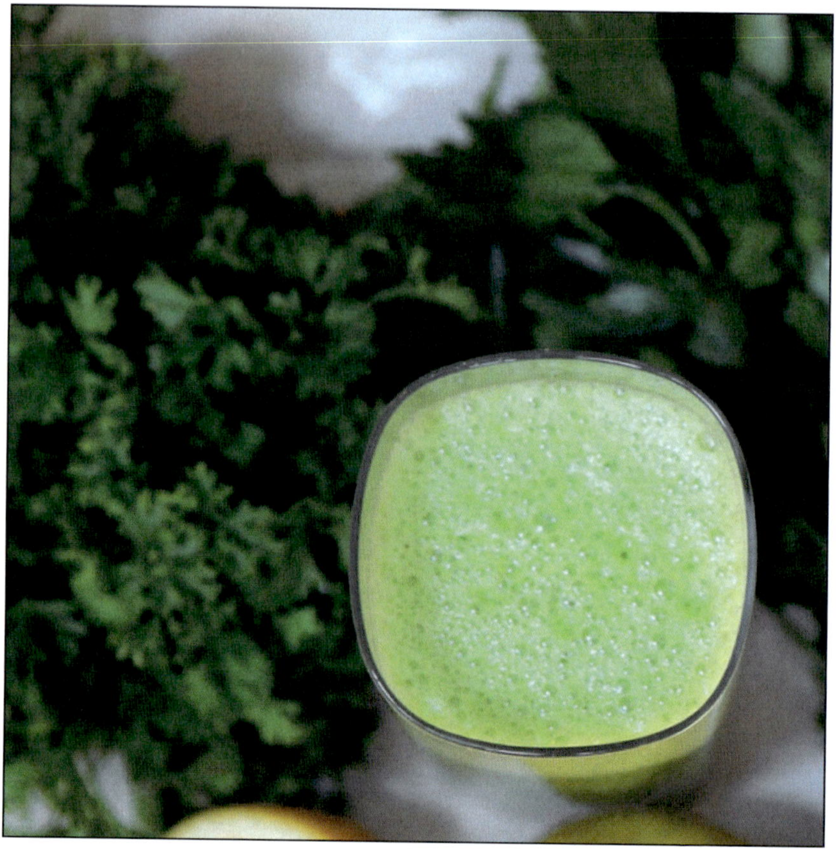

Herbs are beautiful, easy to grow, and they're also fantastic additions to just about any smoothie. Here, parsley and arugula combine to act as a natural diuretic and help to relieve bloating. Parsley also has antibacterial and antifungal qualities. The sweetness of the apples masks any bitterness imparted by the greens, although this is not a sweet smoothie. It has a lovely, refreshing, grassy quality.

Ingredients

- 1 cup arugula, loosely packed
- 1 cucumber
- 2 apples, seeded and quartered
- 1 stalk celery
- ½ cup parsley, loosely packed. Start with a little and add more to taste.
- 1 cup ice

Your Notes

12. Dandelion Banana Smoothie

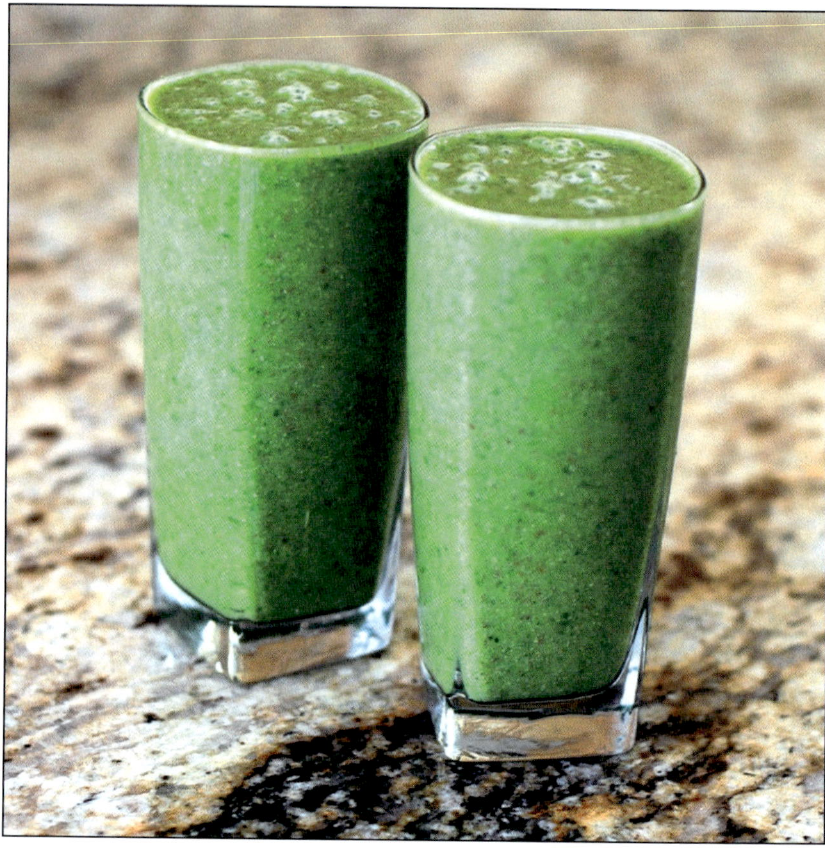

Dandelion greens are sold now in many grocery stores. Look for leaves that are green and firm, not wilting and discolored. Add any unused dandelion greens to a phenomenal salad that is certain to surprise your guests.

Ingredients

- 1 cup dandelion greens
- 2 bananas
- 1 orange, peeled and seeded
- 1 tbsp. spirulina
- 1 cup ice

Your Notes

13. Tahini Fig Smoothie

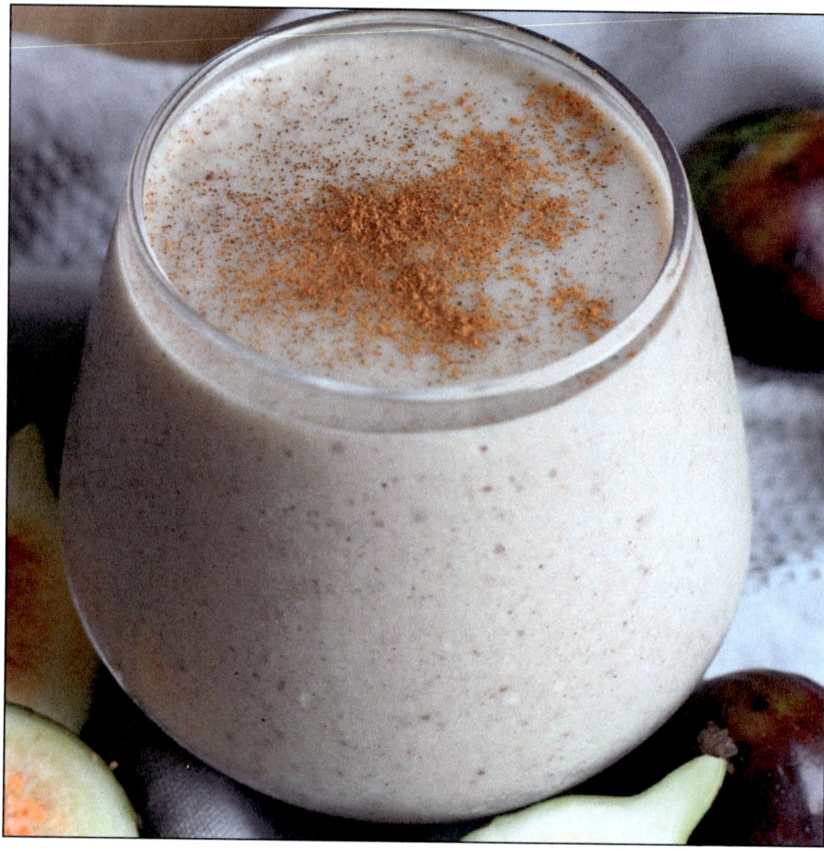

Tahini is a Middle Eastern paste made from ground sesame seeds. It is incredibly versatile, lending its nutty richness to everything from salad dressings to cookies. It can enhance both sweet and savory foods. I keep a jar in my fridge at all times. Here, the tahini serves as a nut butter substitute, delivering vitamin E and B2, along with lots of calcium.

Ingredients

- 1 cup spinach
- Several figs
- 1 apple, seeded and quartered
- 2 tbsp. tahini
- 3 tbsp. chia seeds
- 1 cup ice

Your Notes

14. Almond Butter & Blueberry Elixir

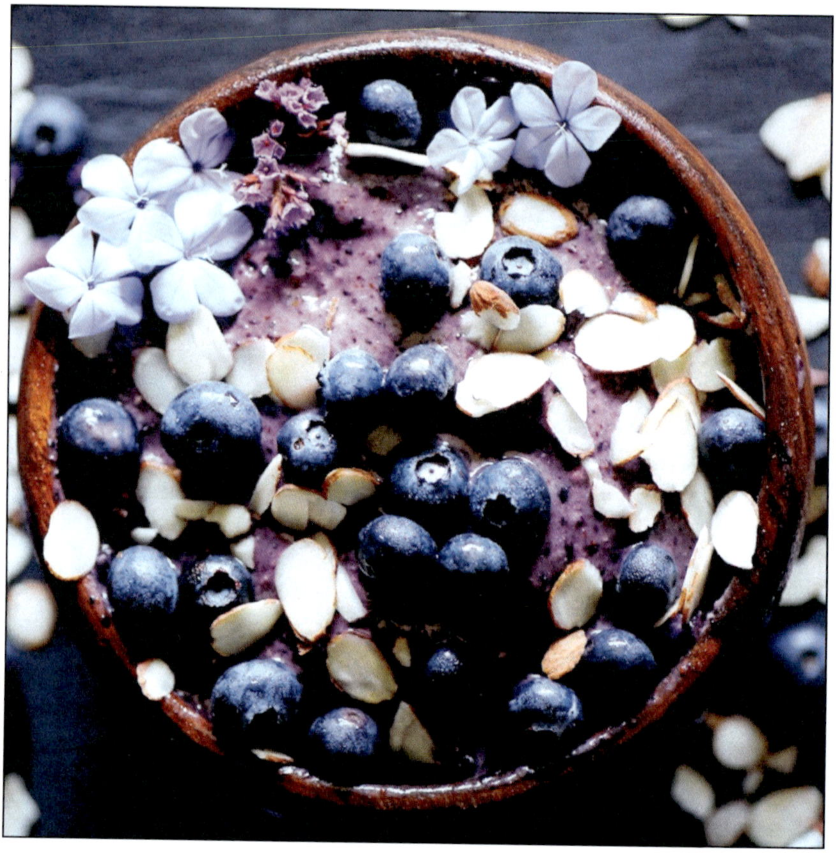

Almond butter is primarily composed of healthy monounsaturated fats, which are effective for lowering cholesterol and high blood pressure levels. Additionally, almond butter is a great source of antioxidants and vitamin E, which are important for the prevention of premature aging.

Ingredients

- 1 cup unsweetened almond milk (or water)
- 1 tbsp. almond butter
- 1 cup blueberries
- 2 cups spinach
- 6 ice cubes
- Top with sliced almonds and blueberries

Your Notes

15. Revitalize & Energize Smoothie

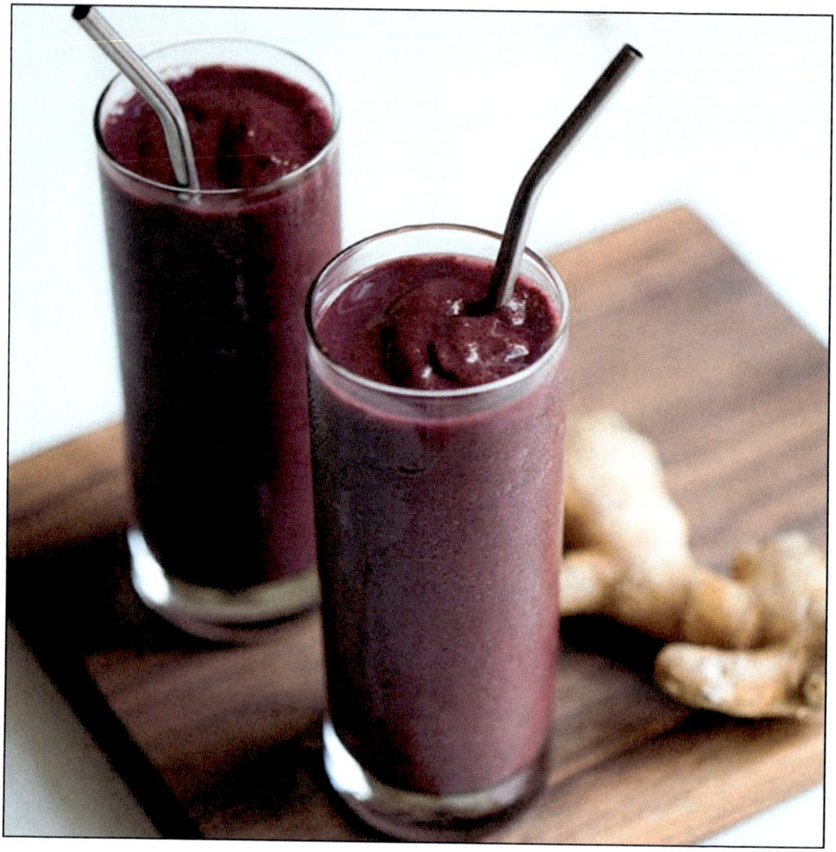

The easy-to-digest carbohydrates in this smoothie will give you sustained energy all day long. Hydration-boosting electrolytes will get you glowing, while blueberries work to cleanse your blood.

Ingredients

- 1-inch piece ginger root, peeled
- 1 cup spinach
- 1 banana
- 1 cup coconut water
- 1 pear (peeled and cored)
- 1 tbsp. hemp seeds
- 1 cup blueberries

Your Notes

16. Cinnamon and Date Smoothie

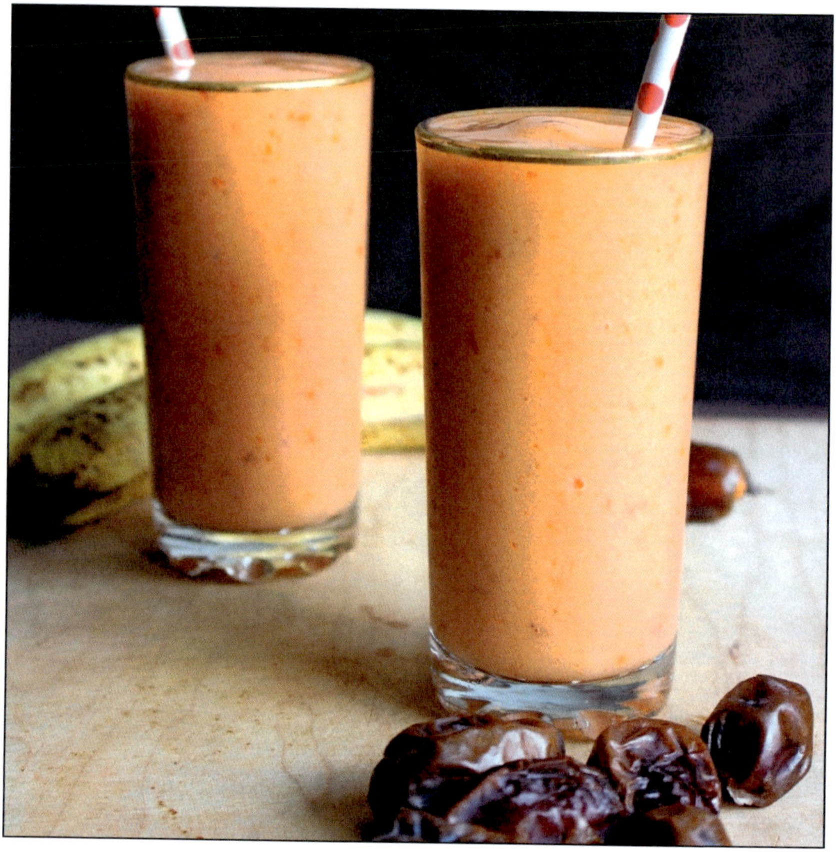

Dates are a great natural source of sweetness, packed with potassium, iron, and magnesium, amongst others. Kale detoxifies and can fight certain cancers with its carotenoids and flavonoids, along with vitamin K.

Ingredients

- 1 apple, seeded & quartered
- 3 Medjool dates, pitted
- 2 kale leaves, ribs removed
- 1 tsp cinnamon powder
- 1 tbsp. hemp or chia seeds
- 1 cup water

Your Notes

17. Collard Greens Smoothie with Chlorella

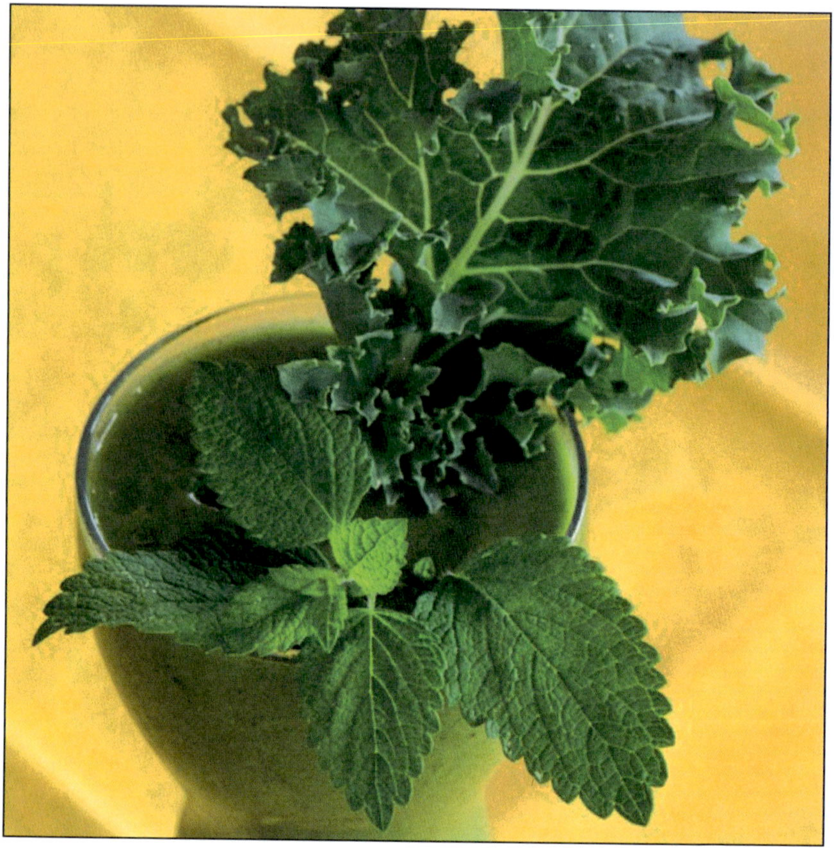

Most people would not think of using collard greens in a smoothie, but they are very healthy for you. Chlorella, a freshwater algae, is the secret boost hidden inside this green smoothie. It is a superfood in every sense of the term, loaded with amino acids, beta-carotene, phosphorous, biotin, and B-complex vitamins.

Ingredients

- 1 cup chopped collard greens
- 2 bananas
- 1 tbsp. parsley
- 1 tbsp. chlorella
- 1 cup ice

Your Notes

18. Dandelion Orange Smoothie

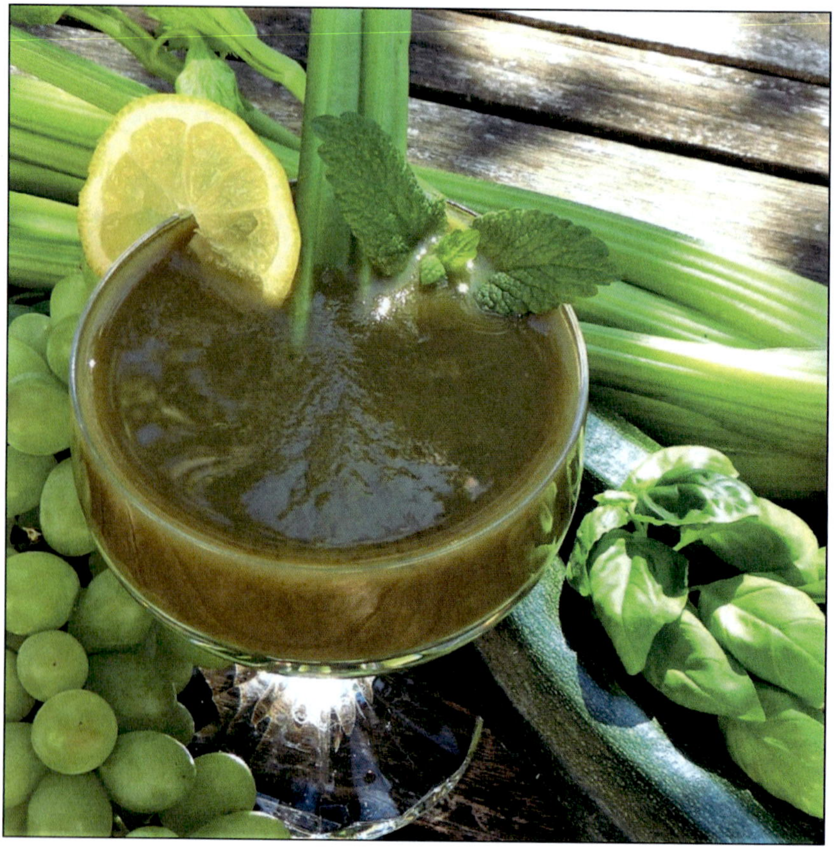

The earthy bitterness of the dandelions enters a happy marriage here with the tart citrus, and creamy avocado. All three flavors meld on the tongue with a bite from the fresh ginger. This will please your palate, and your appetite.

Ingredients

- 1 cup dandelion greens
- 1 orange
- 3/4 avocado
- 1 stalk celery
- 1 tsp. fresh ginger
- 1 cup ice

Your Notes

19. Triple A Smoothie

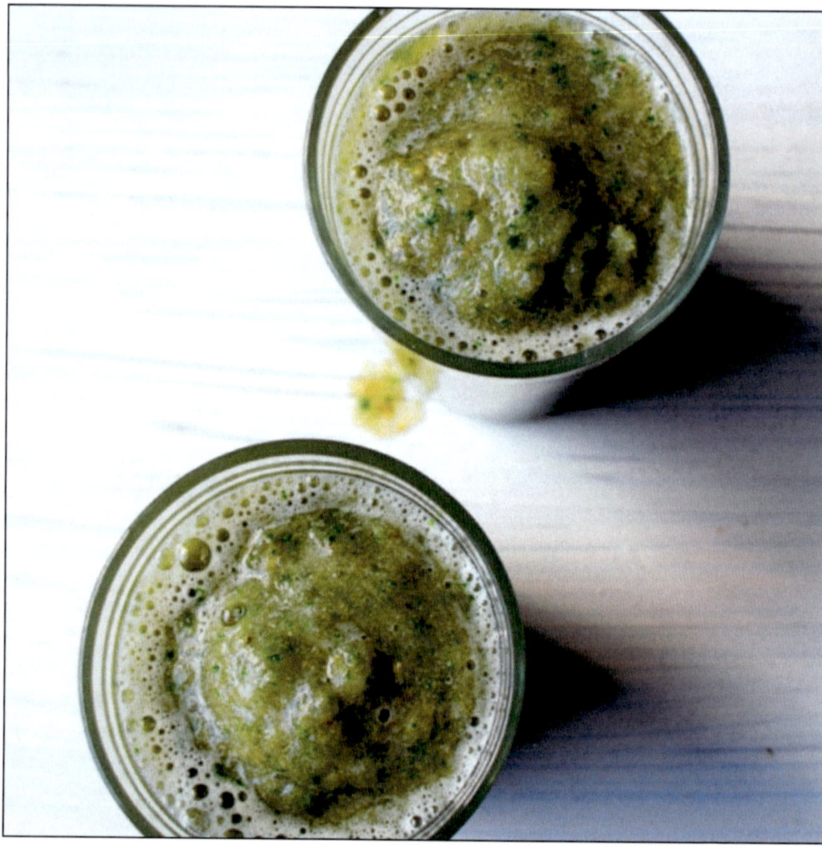

The peppery taste of arugula is balanced by the sweetness of the apple; and the nuttiness of the almond butter smoothes out this trio.

Ingredients

- 1 cup arugula
- 2 apples, seeded and quartered
- 2 tbsp. natural almond butter
- 1 tbsp. chia seeds
- 1 cup ice

Your Notes

20. Barley Grass Smoothie

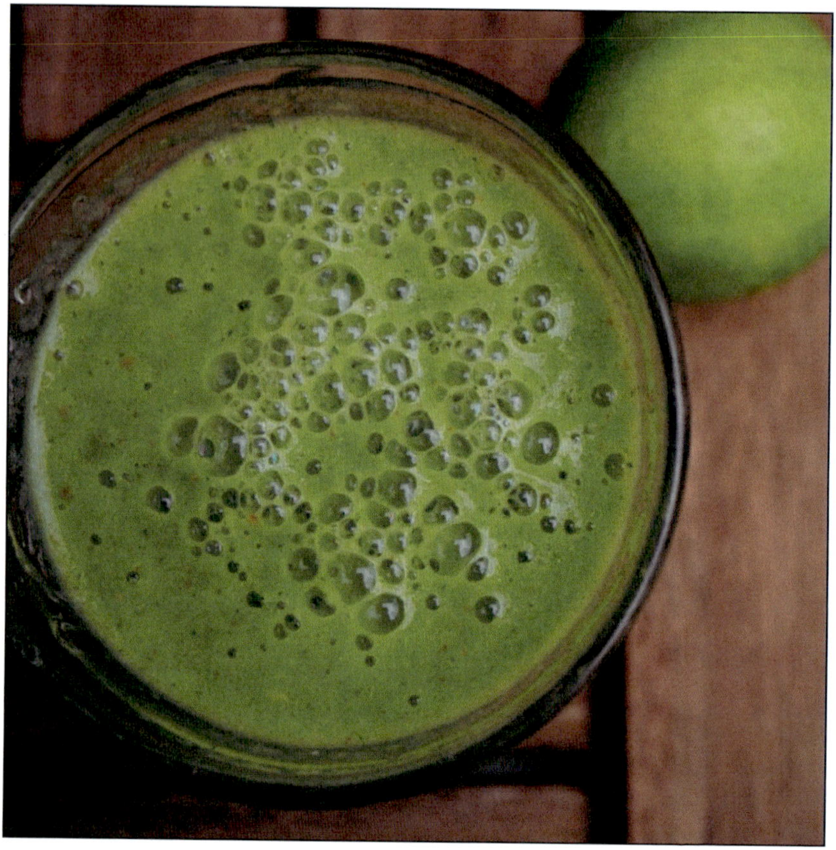

You probably know of barley, the ancient grain, but have you heard of barley grass? The young shoots of the barley plant are harvested and can be juiced just like wheatgrass. It also comes in powder form. However you consume it, you will benefit from its many minerals, including calcium, iron, potassium, and magnesium. It also contains an enzyme that can demolish free radicals that harm the body.

Ingredients

- 1 cup barley grass
- 2 bananas
- 1 tbsp. cilantro
- 1/4 lime, peel included
- 1 tsp. spirulina
- 1 cup ice

Your Notes

21. Bee Pollen Cauliflower Smoothie

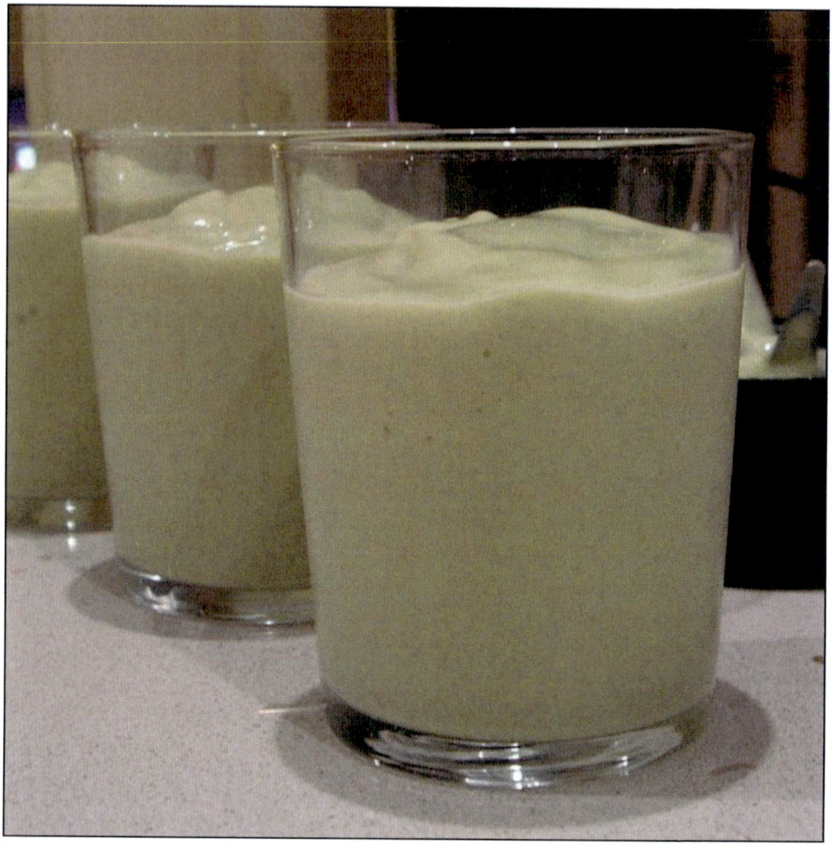

Bee pollen is always in my pantry. This superfood derived from the honey-making process does everything from strengthening the immune system to lowering cholesterol. You'll also love cauliflower as a smoothie ingredient: It creates a creamy texture while allowing stronger flavors to shine. The pinch of nutmeg takes this smoothie to a whole new flavor level.

Ingredients

- 1 cup cauliflower florets
- 3 kiwis
- 1 banana
- 1 tbsp. bee pollen
- 1 cup ice
- Pinch of nutmeg

Your Notes

22. Mango Cantaloupe Smoothie

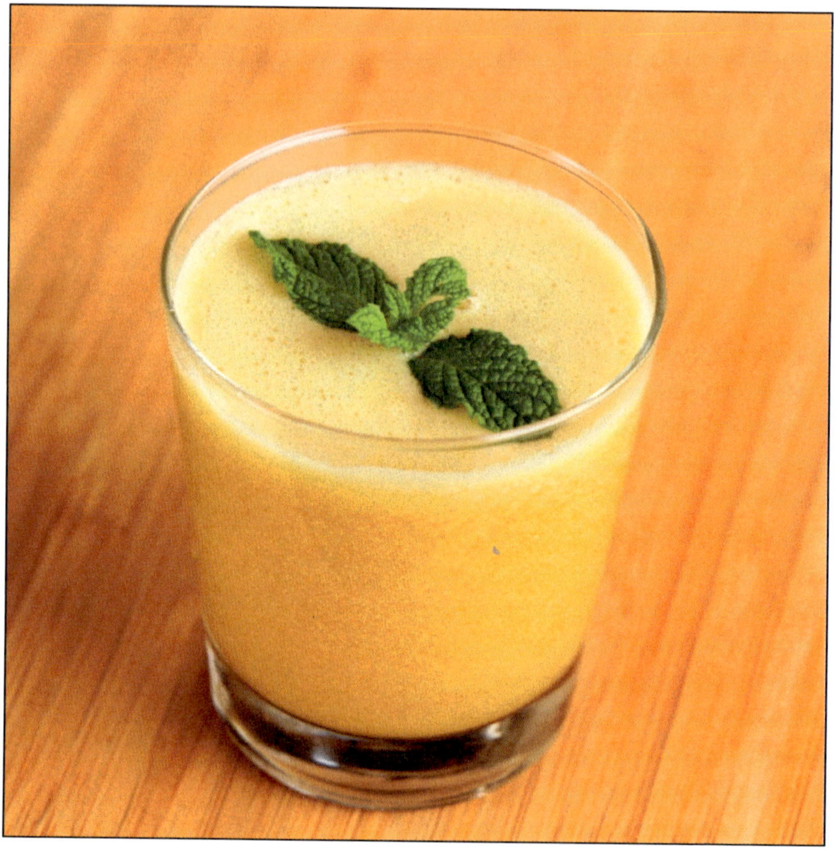

There are few things more fantastic than a good mango smoothie. This tropical fruit was born to be blended. Maqui berry powder is also an antioxidant powerhouse, containing an estimated 10x the amount in acai berries. If you're purchasing this powder online, look for raw, organic selections.

Ingredients

- 1 cup cantaloupe
- 1 mango, peeled and seeded
- 3 kiwis
- 1 tbsp. tahini
- 1 tbsp. maqui berry powder
- 1 cup ice

Your Notes

23. Pumpkin Grapefruit Smoothie

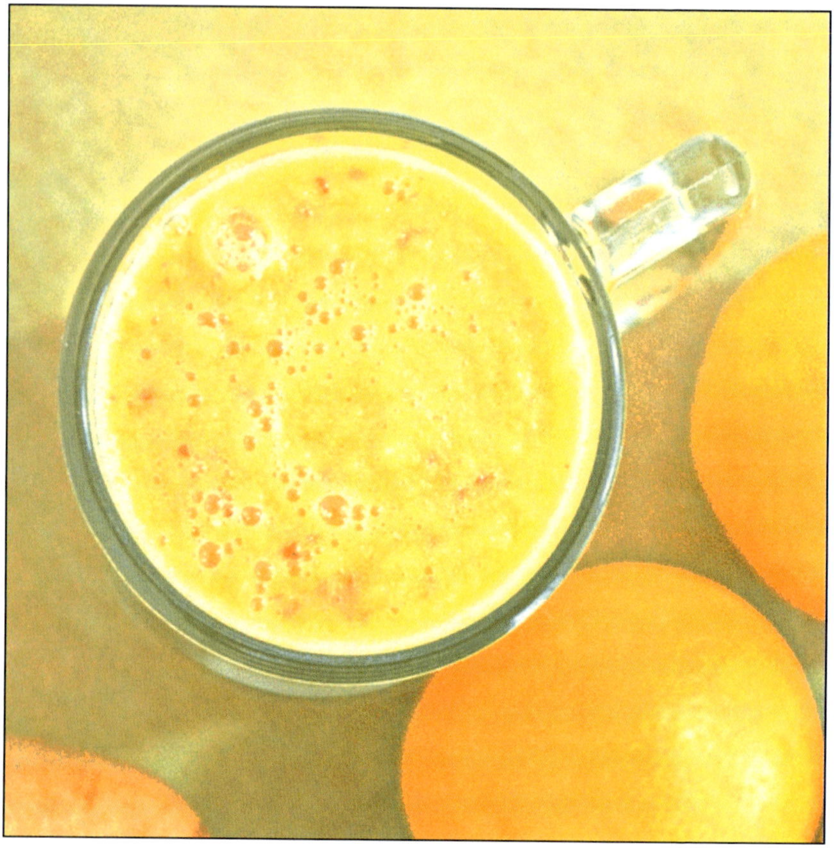

We treat pumpkin as a seasonal gourd, but this smoothie is truly accessible all year round. Organic pumpkin is now available both in cans, and frozen. Just don't pick up any "pumpkin filling" junk on accident—pumpkin should be the only ingredient. I will admit, this smoothie does remind me of fall. The citrus, pumpkin and ginger combination imparts warmth. I like to sprinkle a little cinnamon on top.

Ingredients

- 1 cup pumpkin
- 1 mango, peeled and seeded
- 1 grapefruit, peeled and seeded
- 1 tbsp. fresh ginger
- 1 tbsp. tahini
- 1 cup ice

Your Notes

24. Matcha-Berry Green Smoothie

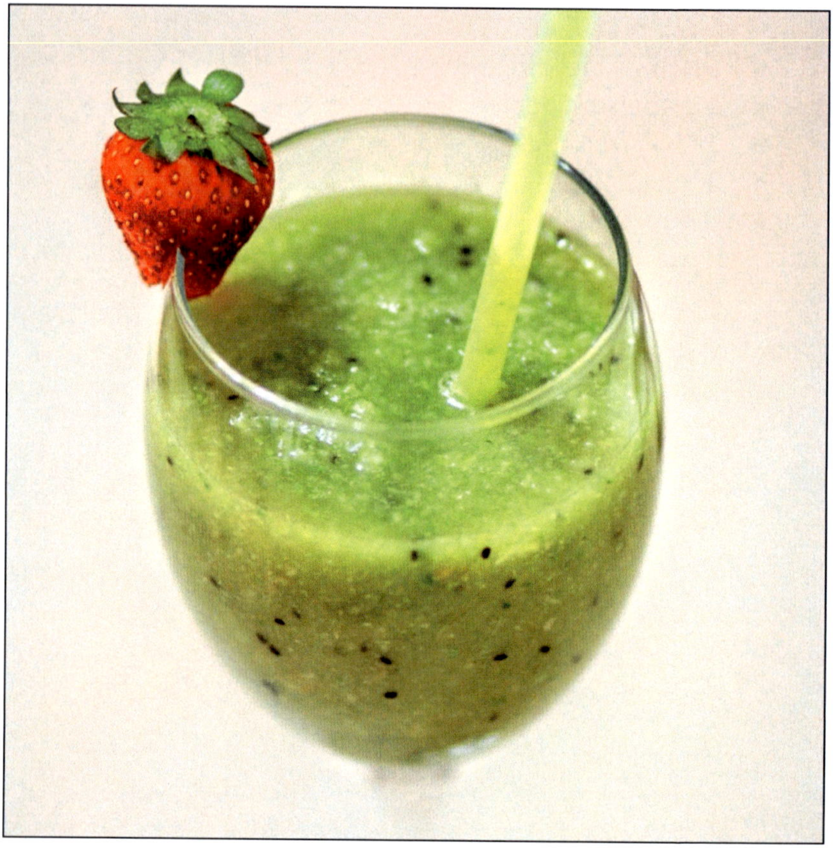

Matcha is rich in antioxidants, has free radical-scavenging activity and encourages your body's natural detoxification systems. If you keep sliced bananas in your freezer for your smoothie stash, you won't need to use ice!

Ingredients

- ½ cup mixed berries
- 1 frozen sliced banana
- 1 tsp. Matcha powder
- ½ cup almond milk
- ½ cup ice

Your Notes

25. Coconut Spirulina Smoothie

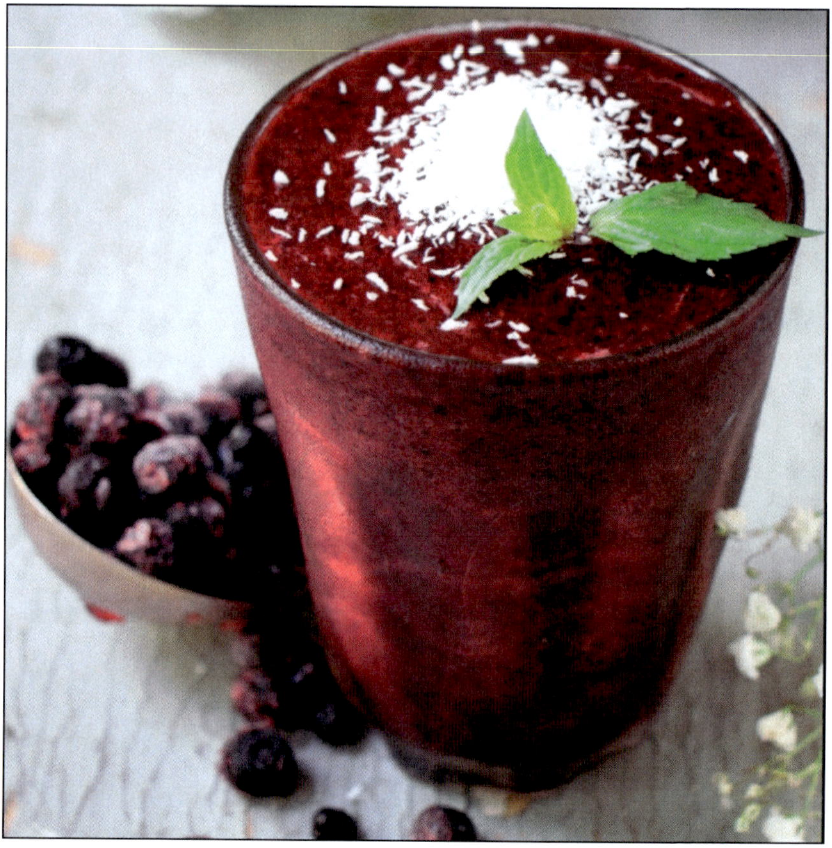

The Coconut Spirulina Smoothie is a smorgasbord of superfoods. On top of the berry-banana-greens base, maca powder and spirulina powder combine to boost your energy, immune system, mood, and memory.

Ingredients

- 1 banana
- ½ cup blueberries
- 1 cup baby spinach
- ½ cup kale, ribs removed
- 1 tbsp. honey
- 1 tbsp. maca powder
- 1 tbsp. spirulina powder
- ¼ tsp. cinnamon
- 1 ½ cup coconut milk

Your Notes

26. Coconut Milk Green Dandelion Smoothie

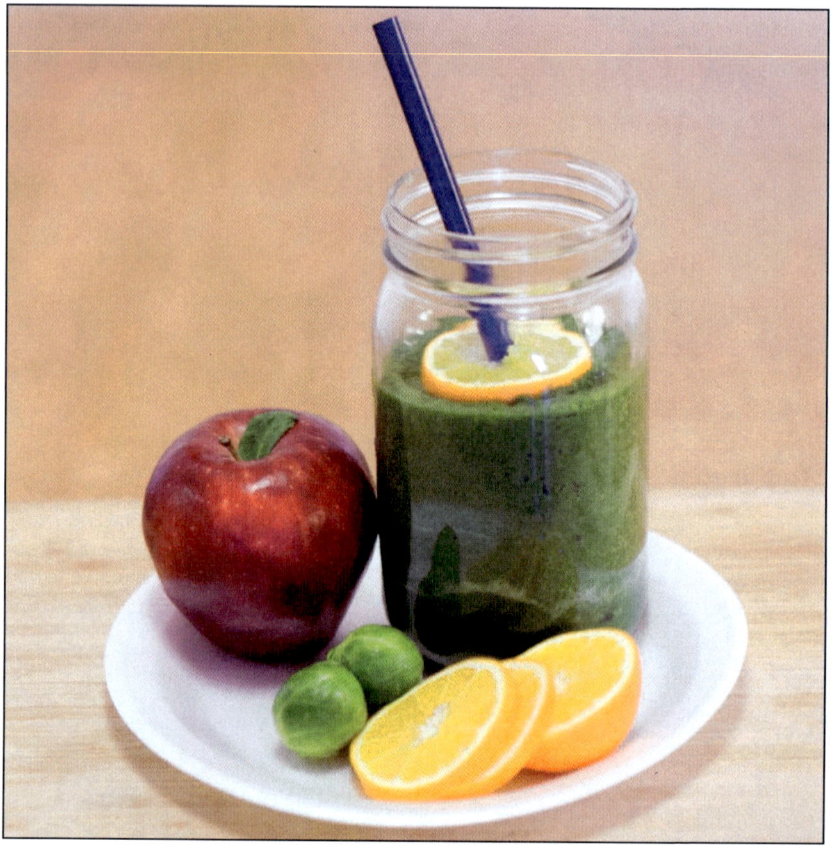

With all my smoothies, I like to experiment and try new combinations and variations. This smoothie was designed to accommodate virtually any superfood supplement, although it's also a killer drink without anything added. I also sometimes throw in some pith and peel of the lemon for an added citrus zing. It's fantastic.

Ingredients

- 1 apple, seeded and quartered
- 1 banana
- 1 cup dandelion greens
- Juice of 1 lemon
- 1 cup coconut milk

Your Notes

27. Spinach Spirulina Smoothie

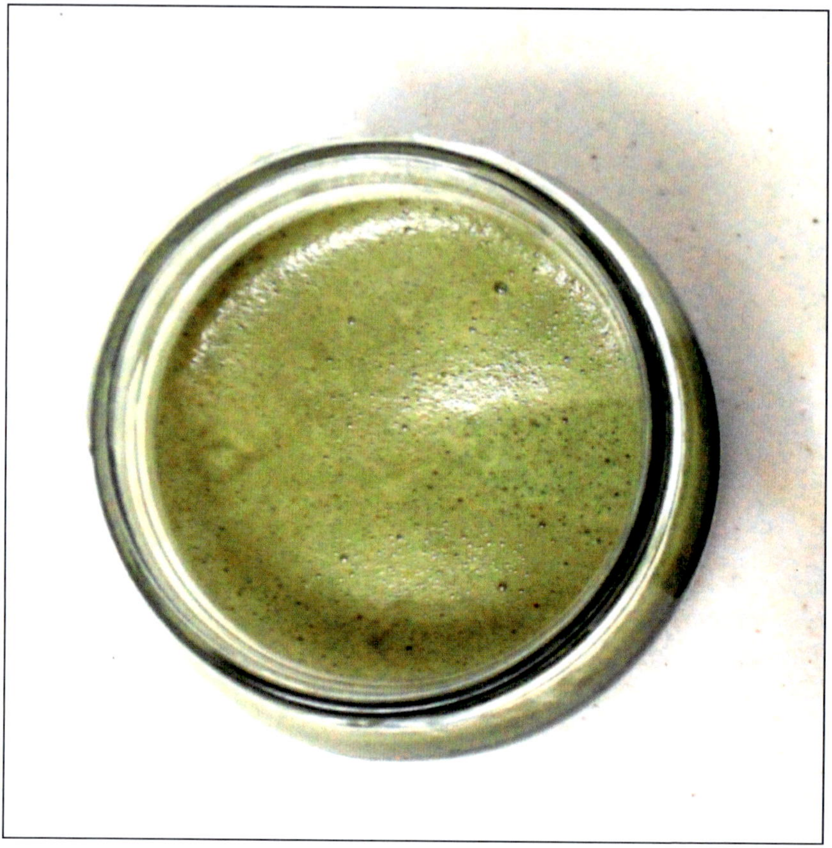

Spirulina has an admittedly less-than-wonderful taste, which is why a smoothie is the ideal vehicle for delivering its powerful punch. Its added fiber and protein is a tool in the fight for weight loss. It can aid in reducing inflammation, and has antimicrobial properties, such as helping with candida infections in the mouth, gut, and vagina.

Ingredients

- 2 cups baby spinach
- 1 banana
- 2 tsp spirulina
- 1 tbsp. maple syrup
- 1 cup almond milk

Your Notes

28. Green Kiwi Flax Smoothie

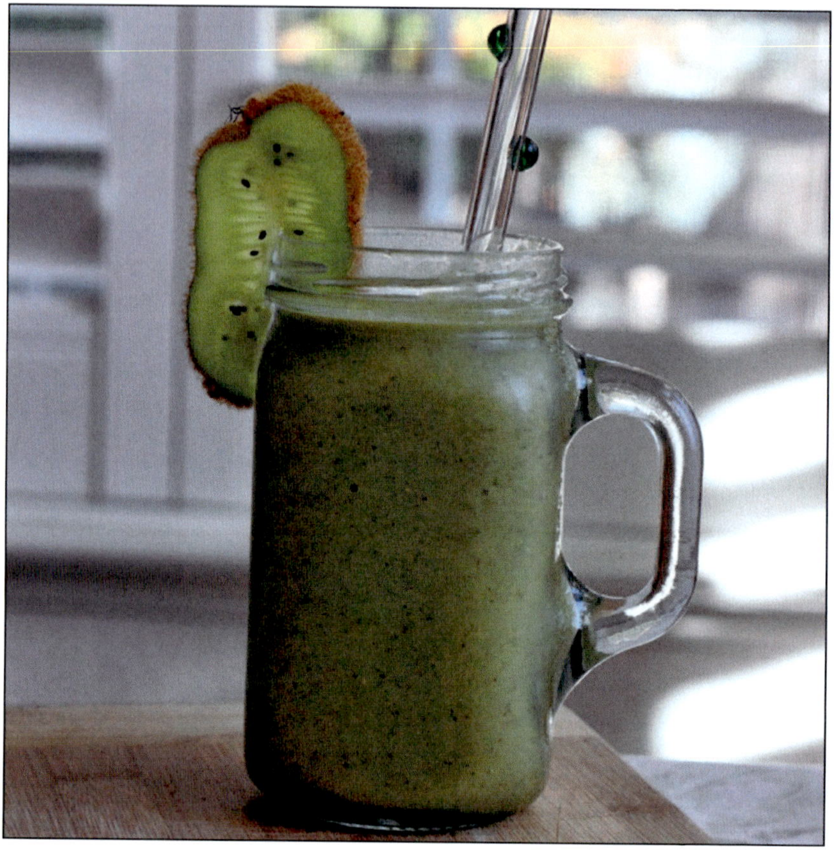

Aside from their sweet and tangy flesh, kiwis also boast high antioxidant and vitamins C, K, and E levels. Here is a little-known fact—kiwi skin is completely edible, so don't waste your time peeling them for smoothies. Just toss them right in and you will increase the nutrient density!

Ingredients

- 2 cups baby spinach
- 2 kiwis
- 1 banana
- 1 tbsp. ground flaxseed
- ½ cup water
- ½ cup ice

Your Notes

29. Honey Banana Green Smoothie

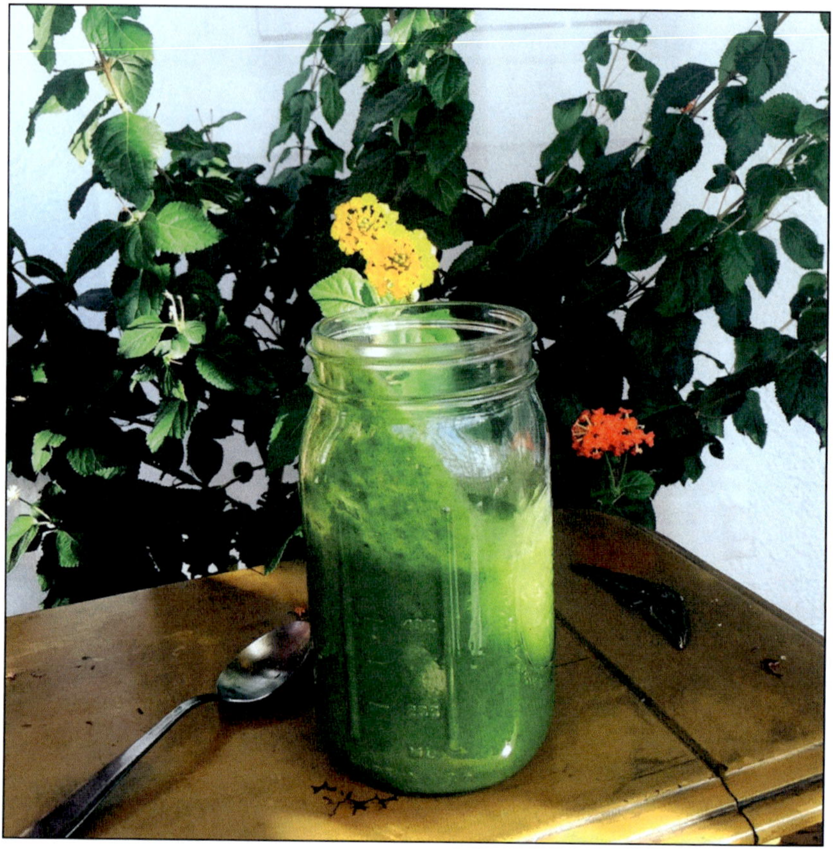

This smoothie is actually just as great a face mask as it is a drink. Internal benefits include clearer skin, lots of omega-3's, and tons of fiber. Vegans can sub maple syrup or lucuma powder for the honey.

Ingredients

- 2 cups baby spinach
- 1 green apple
- 1 banana
- 2 tsp honey
- 1 tsp spirulina
- 1 tbsp. ground flaxseed
- ½ cup water
- ½ cup ice

Your Notes

30. Green Goji Berry Smoothie

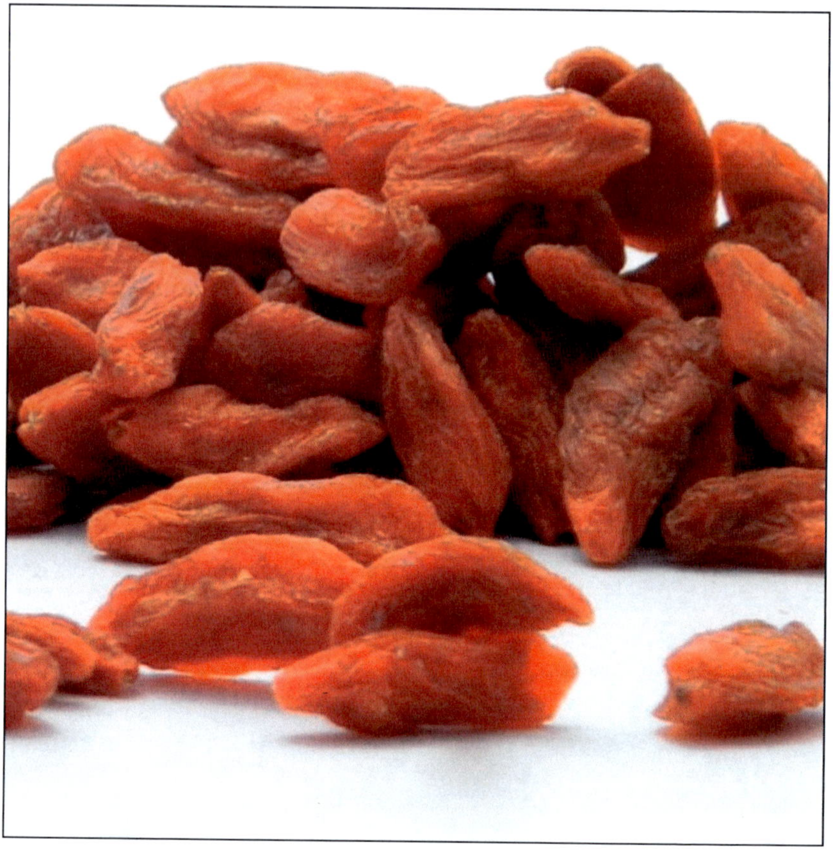

Low in calories and fat-free, dried Goji berries can be tossed on top of virtually anything. I like to pile them on oatmeal, add them to salads, and they're a top 5 acai bowl topping. I'm blessed to actually own a goji plant. Here, the Goji berries bring additional antioxidant power and gastrointestinal healing to a truly healthy beverage.

Ingredients

- 1 cup kale, ribs removed
- ½-cup Goji berries
- 1 green apple, seeded and quartered
- 2 tbsp. flaxseeds
- 2 tsp honey
- 2 cups water

Your Notes

31. Almond Cashew Smoothie

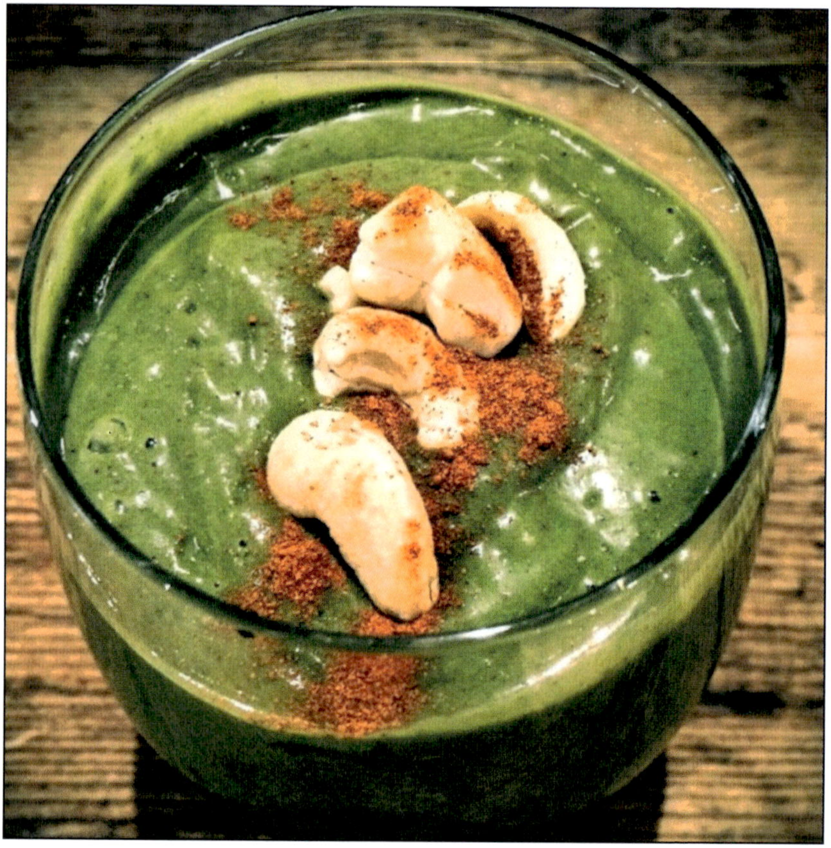

Go nuts with the fantastic combo of almond milk and softened cashews. While soaking is not required, I'd recommend doing it for at least an hour because ingredients will blend together much better. You may already know that cashews are packed with healthy fats, but did you know that they rock lots of essential minerals too? Not only that, they are a protein powerhouse.

Ingredients

- 1 cup spinach
- 1 cup cashews, soaked overnight
- 1 tbsp. agave nectar
- 1 tsp vanilla extract
- 1 cup unsweetened almond milk
- 1 cup ice

Your Notes

32. Watermelon Moringa Smoothie

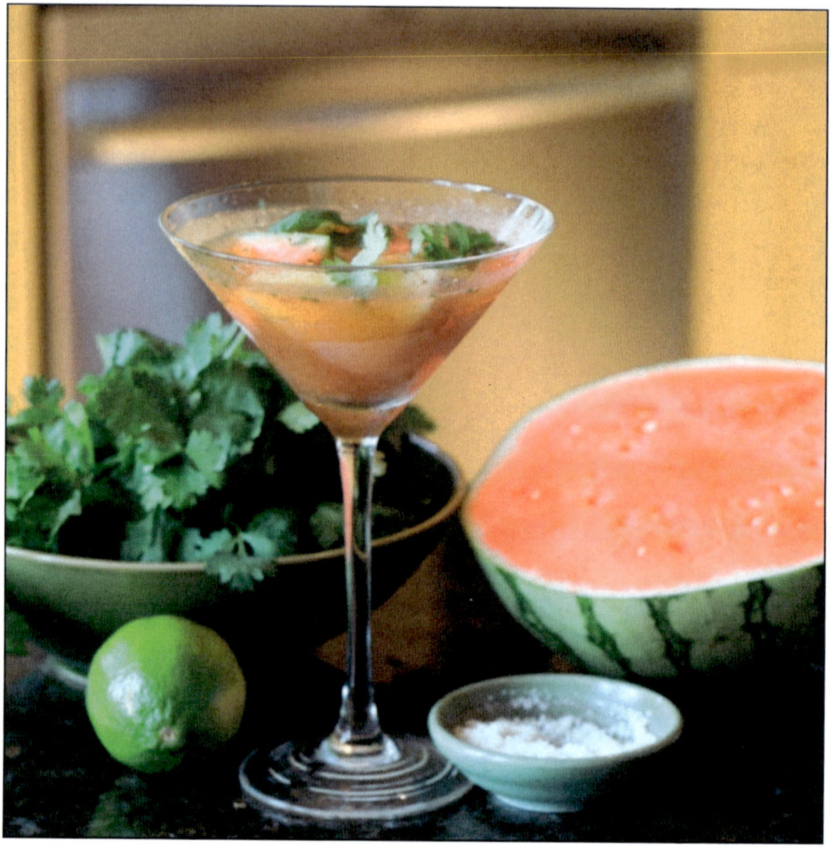

Moringa powder has its own delicious spinach-y flavor, and does wonders in a morning smoothie. You will benefit from its 9 amino acids, fiber, iron, vitamin K and calcium. It is another highly bioavailable supplement worth keeping in your kitchen at all times.

Ingredients

- ½ cup water
- ¾ cup red grapes
- 1 ripe banana
- ½ cup of kale
- ½ cup watermelon
- 1 tbsp. moringa powder
- ¼ cup ice

Your Notes

33. Strawberry Energy Smoothie

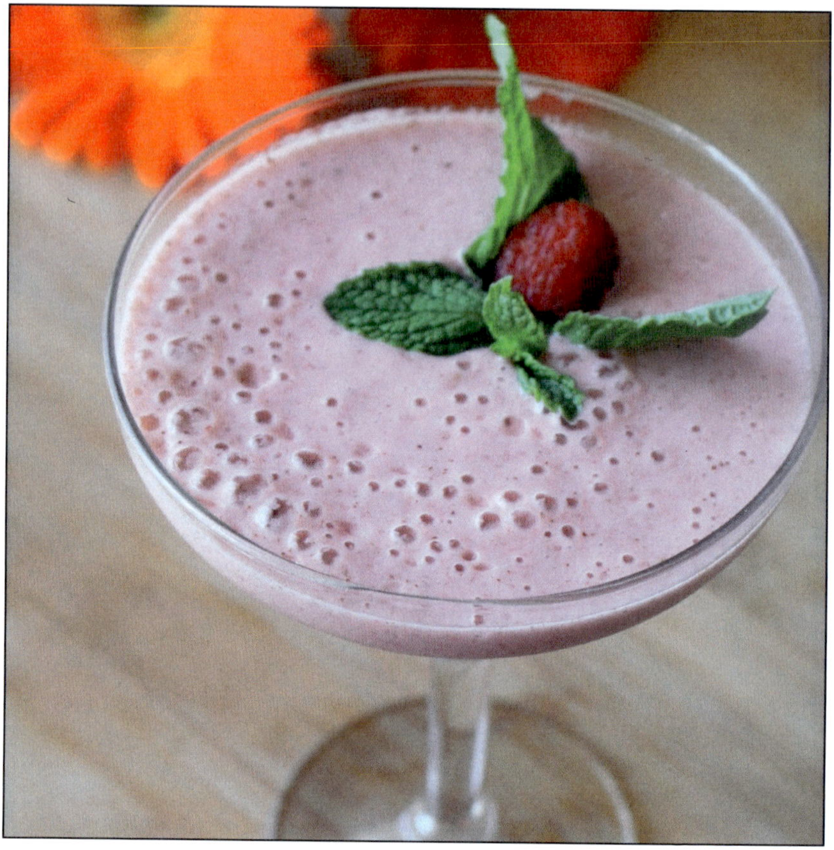

I don't think there are any smoothie ingredients more universally delicious than the common strawberry. When combined with a solid kick of ginger, both flavors are elevated. If you want to take the Strawberry Energy Smoothie up another notch, I highly recommend coconut milk to replace the water.

Ingredients

- 1 cup strawberries
- 1 apple, seeded & quartered
- 1 inch fresh ginger, peeled
- 1 tsp. moringa powder
- 1 cup water

Your Notes

34. Avocado Berry Smoothie

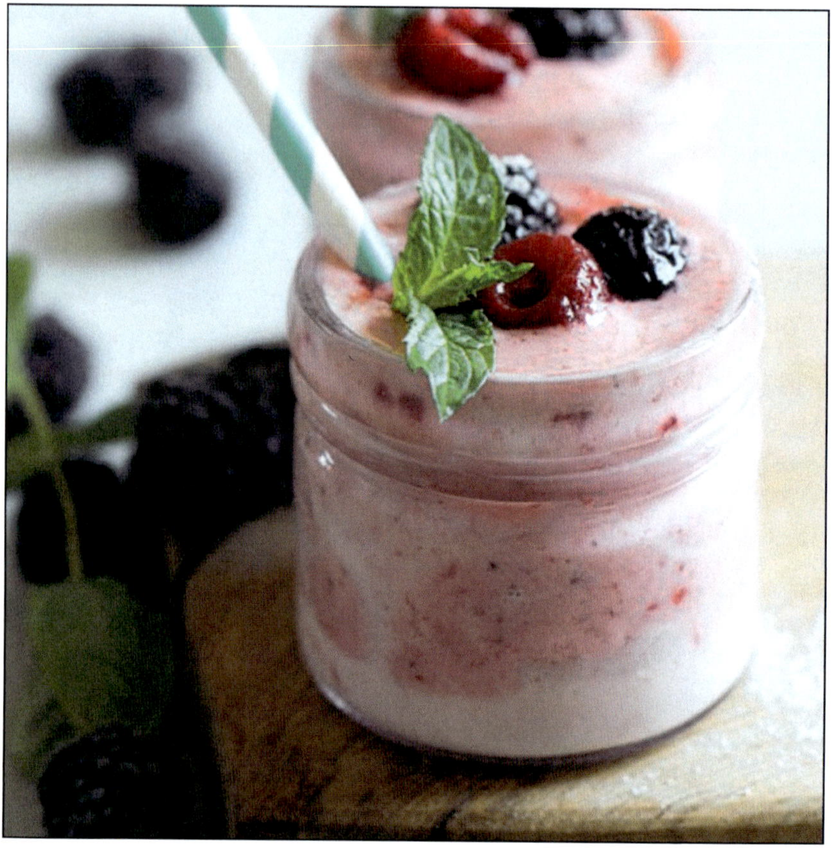

Moringa powder is a quick way to deliver fiber, iron, vitamins and amino acids straight to your system every morning. When it is combined with berries, mango and avocado, you get one of the best-tasting drinks around.

Ingredients

- ½ cup water
- ½ cup raspberries
- ½ cup blueberries
- ½ cup mango
- 1/2 avocado
- ½ cup ice
- 1 tbsp moringa powder

Your Notes

35. Blackberry Comfort Smoothie

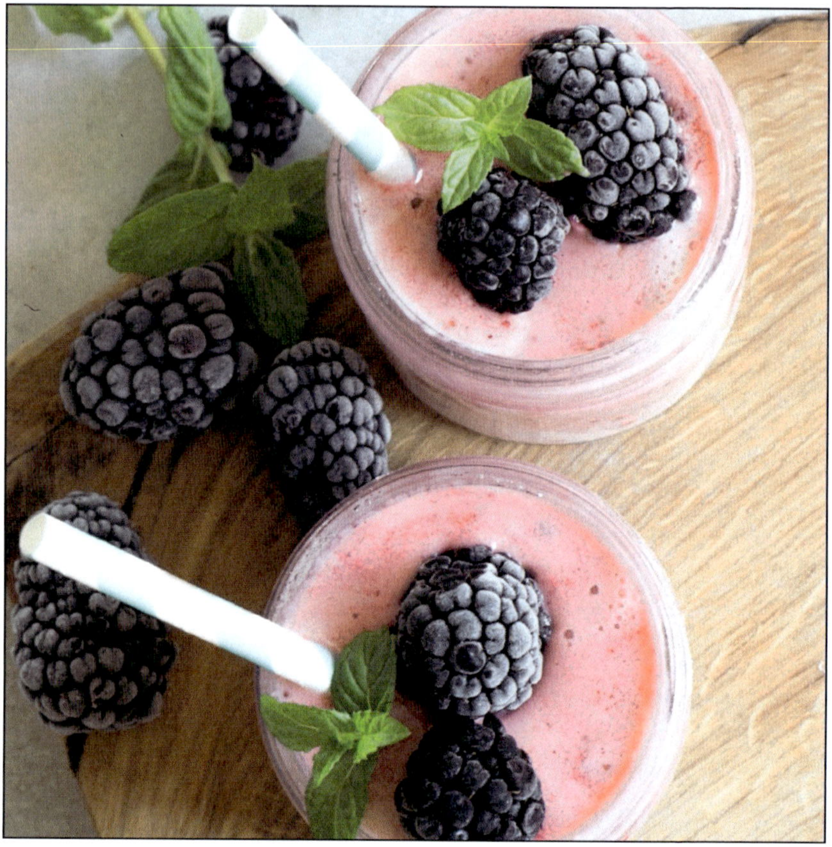

When blackberries are in season, I go nuts trying to include them in everything – they are that good. They deliver antioxidants in spades, just like the moringa powder. The creaminess of the mango and the almond milk base turn this into a truly comforting beverage.

Ingredients

- ½ cup blackberries
- ½ cup spinach
- ½ cup mango
- 1 cup unsweetened almond milk
- ¼ tsp vanilla extract
- 1 tbsp. moringa powder
- 2-3 ice cubes

Your Notes

36. Orange Pineapple Smoothie

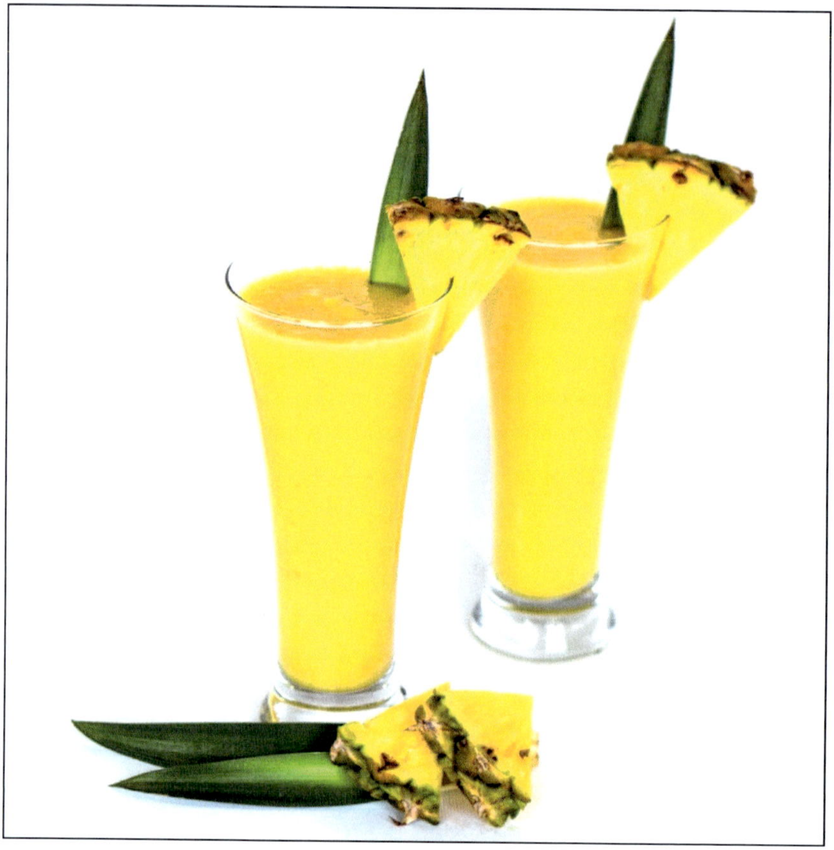

The 1-2 punch of oranges and pineapples is hard to beat. Here, I've layered these tropical beauties with moringa powder to increase vitamin A and calcium levels, along with iron. Because vitamin A increases the uptake of that natural iron into your system, you will feel an almost immediate energy gain.

Ingredients

- ½ cup water
- 1 ripe banana
- 1 orange, peeled and seeded
- 1 cup pineapple
- ½ cup spinach
- 1 tbsp. moringa powder

Your Notes

37. Peachy Bliss Smoothie

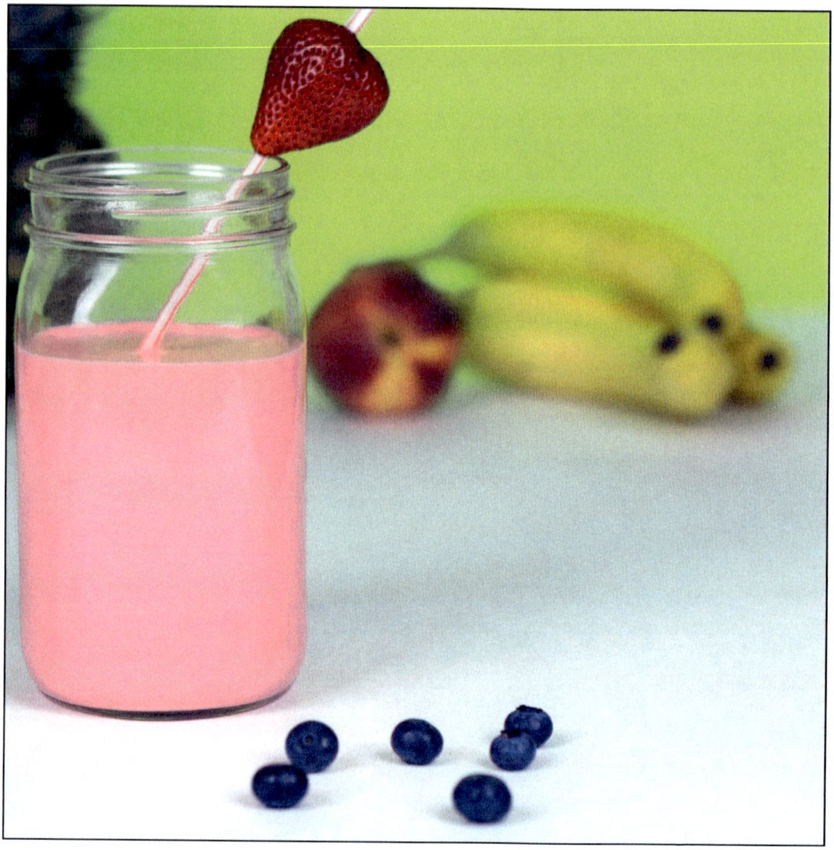

Any berry blends well with the peach in this smoothie! A banana also works well.

Ingredients

- 1 cup blueberries
- 1 peach, pitted & chopped (may substitute frozen peaches too)
- ½ cup spinach
- ½ cup unsweetened almond milk
- 1 tbsp. moringa powder

Your Notes

38. Pineberry Smoothie

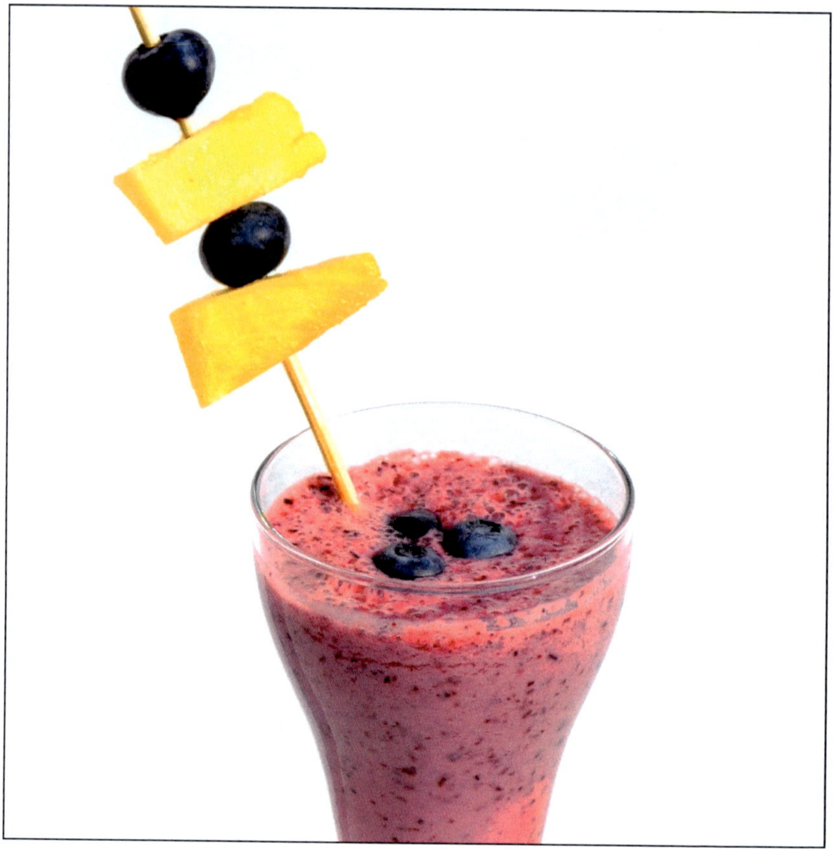

After you've tried pineapple juice in a smoothie, you'll wonder how you ever used anything else. Keep a berry stock in the freezer at all times, and you won't have to grab ice cubes for fruity drinks every morning. Leave out the spinach for a refreshing afternoon drink.

Ingredients

- ½ cup strawberries
- ½ cup blueberries
- ½ cup pineapple juice
- ¼ cup orange juice
- ½ cup spinach
- 1 tbsp. moringa powder
- ¼ cup ice cubes

Your Notes

39. Almond Raspberry Smoothie

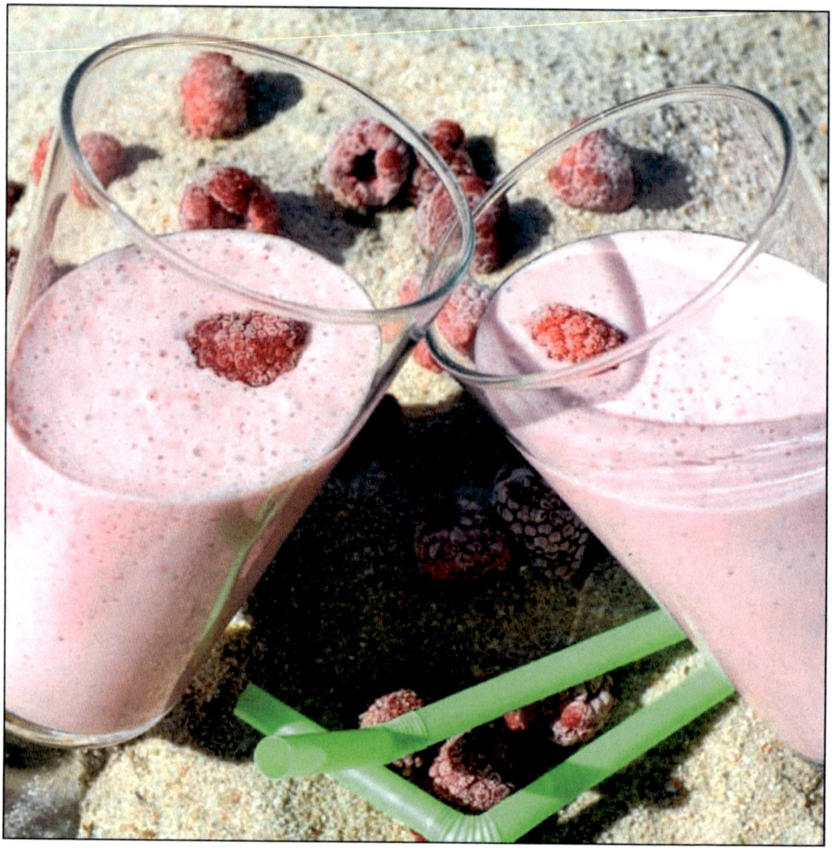

When I ask people if they've incorporated smoothies into their daily routine, I get much of the usual "It's too messy!" or "It takes too much time!" excuses. With this Almond Raspberry Smoothie, those excuses are eliminated. Just 4 ingredients whips together a smoothie with a classic flavor profile, antioxidants, immune system boost, and great energy to get you through to lunch.

Ingredients

- 1 cup unsweetened almond milk
- ½ cup raspberries
- 3 ice cubes
- 1 tbsp. moringa powder

Your Notes

40. Coconut Pineapple Smoothie

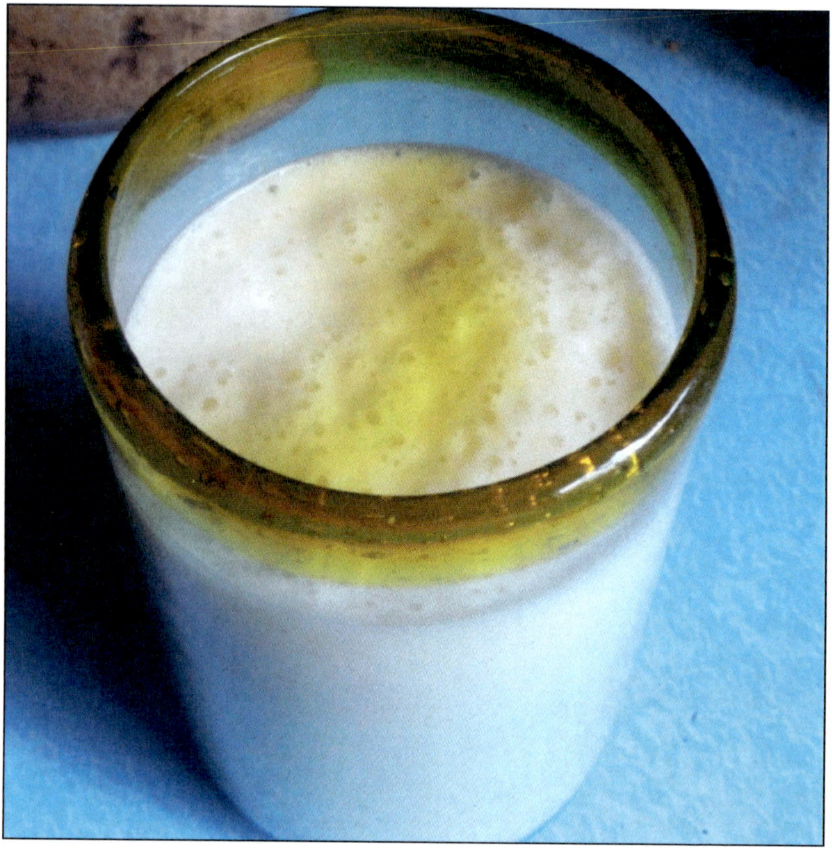

The Coconut Pineapple Smoothie is a dream in a glass. Depending on your healthy fat intake needs, you can now easily find both low-fat and full-fat coconut milk in stores. The wheatgrass powder gives you your green power boost for the day, with amino acids and digestive aid.

Ingredients

- 1 cup coconut milk
- 1 cup pineapple
- 1 tbsp. wheatgrass powder
- 1 cup crushed ice

Your Notes

41. Greek Watermelon Smoothie

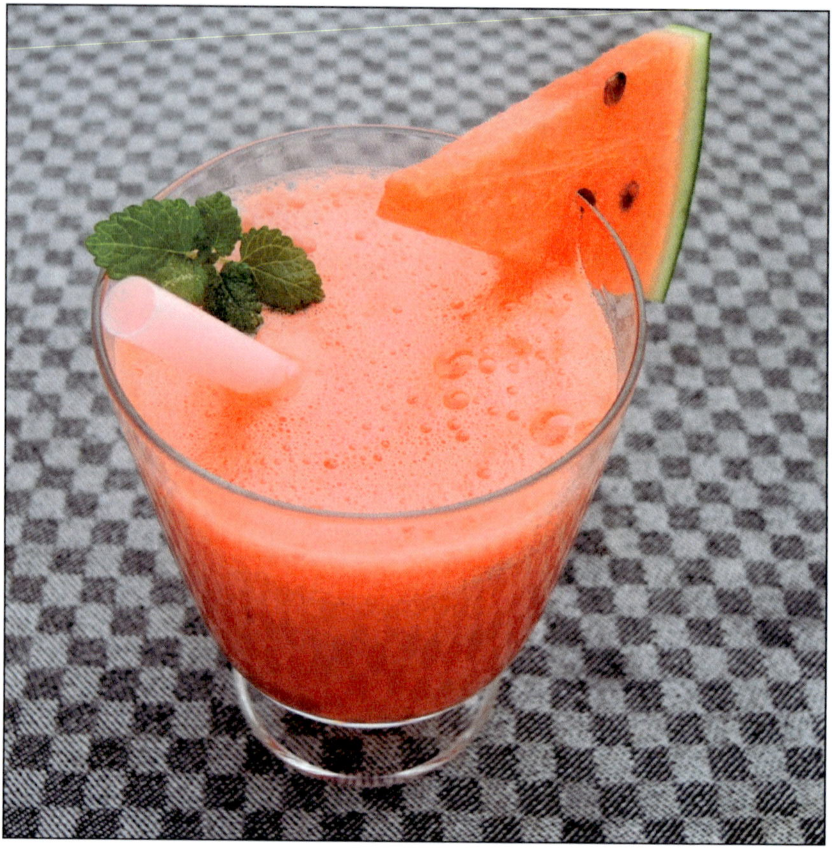

Sail away to the Greek islands with this smoothie inspired by the Mediterranean. The yogurt addition (I prefer coconut milk) gets this shake thick and creamy, while the watermelon hydrates, and the spirulina adds your superfood dose of phytonutrients. Add spinach or kale for more complete nutrition.

Ingredients

- 3 cups seedless watermelon
- 1 cup plain almond milk or coconut milk yogurt
- 1 teaspoon vanilla extract
- 1 teaspoon spirulina
- 1 cup ice

Your Notes

42. Ginger Banana Smoothie with Chlorella

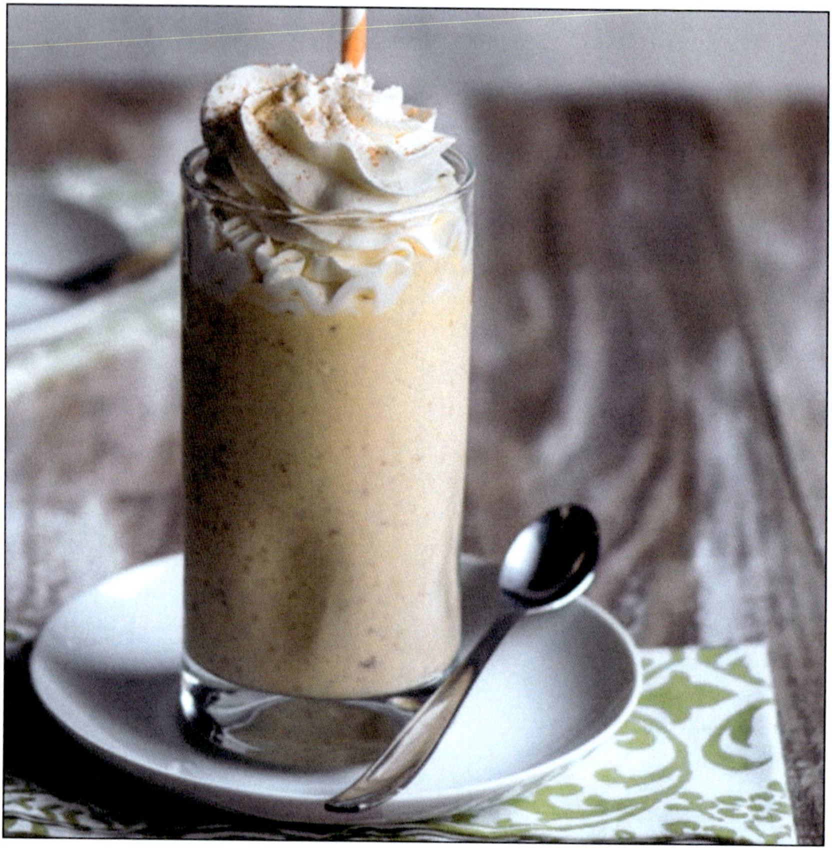

Freshwater algae and other freshwater plants are untapped resources for so many of us. Chlorella contains more than 20 vitamins and minerals, along with more protein than nearly any source found on land.

Ingredients

- 1 banana
- 1 cup unsweetened almond milk
- ½ tsp vanilla extract
- 3 dates, pitted
- ½ tsp ginger, freshly grated
- 1 tsp chlorella

Your Notes

43. Rich Raspberry Matcha Smoothie

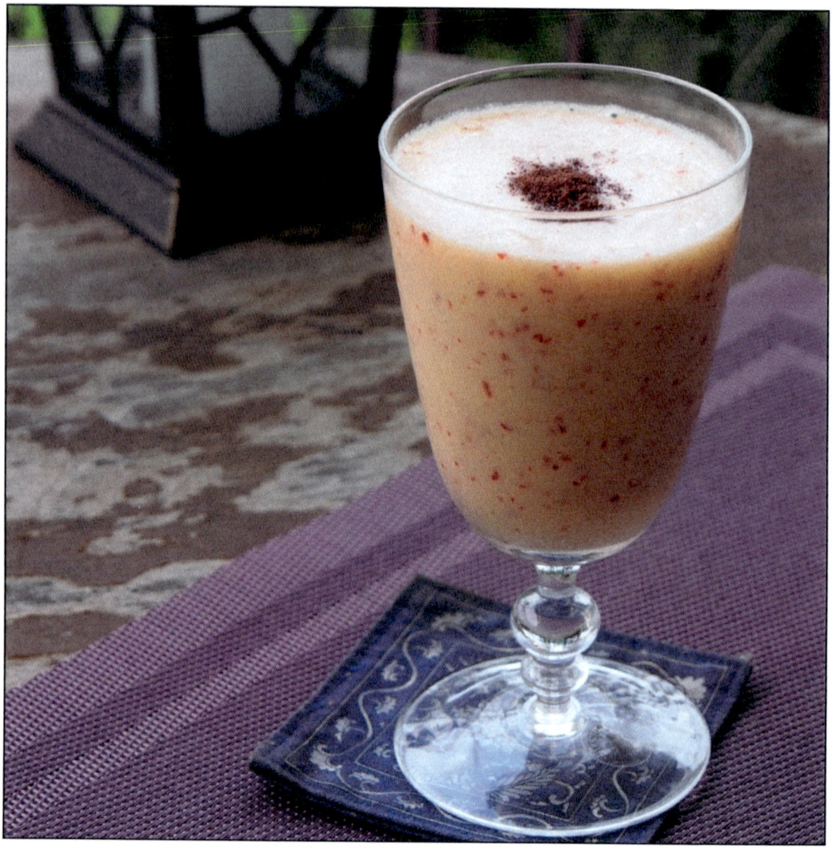

The L-Theanine in Matcha powder gives you the mental focus you crave from coffee and soda drinks without the sugar high and the inevitable drop (also known as the mid-morning slump).

Ingredients

- ¼ cup water
- ¾ cup unsweetened almond milk
- 1 date, pitted
- ¼ cup arugula
- 1½ raspberries
- ½ banana
- 1 tsp Matcha powder

Your Notes

44. Zesty Raspberry Ginger Smoothie

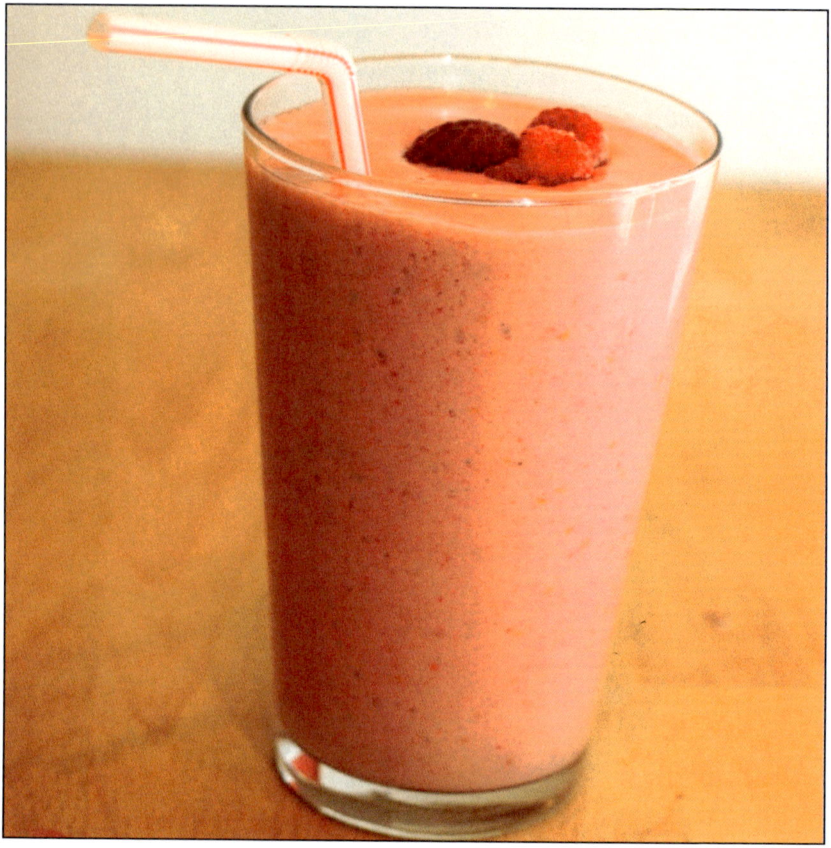

If you could bottle joy, it would probably come with these ingredients. The sweetness of the berries and the dates is balanced out by some freshly-squeezed lemon juice, and then the ginger comes in to leave a tingle on your tongue. The moringa powder adds the finishing superfood touch.

Ingredients

- ½ cup raspberries
- ¾ cup unsweetened almond milk
- ¼ cup strawberries
- 1 tsp ginger, fresh
- 1 tbsp. ground flaxseed
- 1 tsp lemon Juice
- 1 tbsp. moringa powder

Your Notes

45. Espresso Dream Smoothie

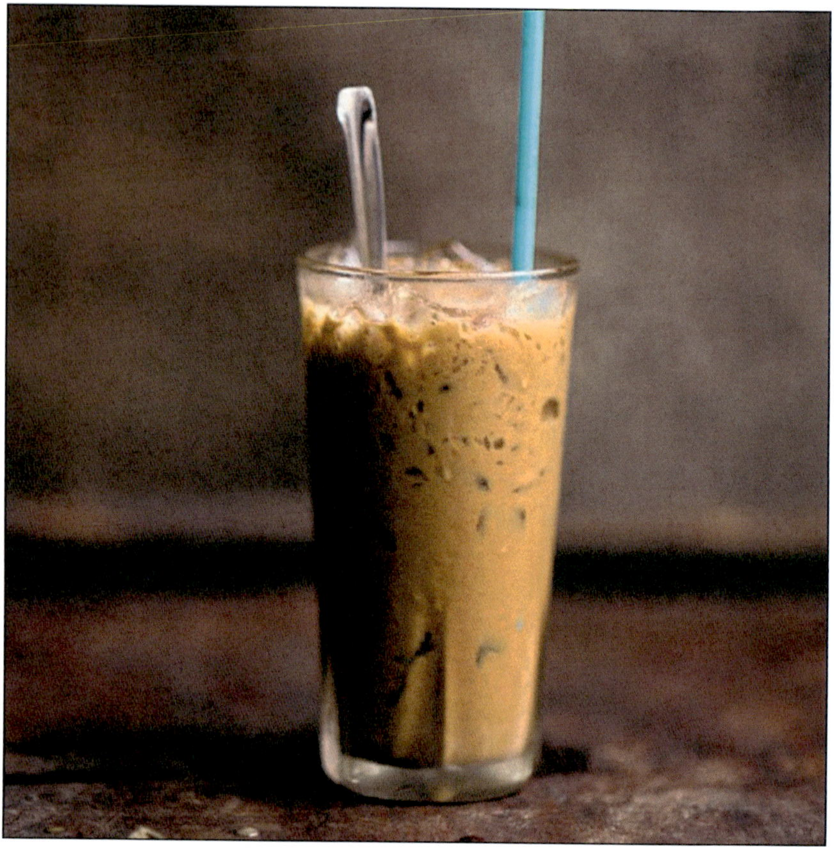

Coffee drinkers don't have to avoid smoothies – the Espresso Dream Smoothie incorporates caffeine to create a drink that rivals any $5 frappe.

Ingredients

- 1 cup unsweetened almond milk
- 1 shot espresso or cold brew coffee
- ¼ cup unsweetened cocoa powder
- 2 tbsp. agave nectar
- ½ cup ice
- 1 tbsp. moringa powder

Your Notes

46. Healthy Peanut Butter Smoothie

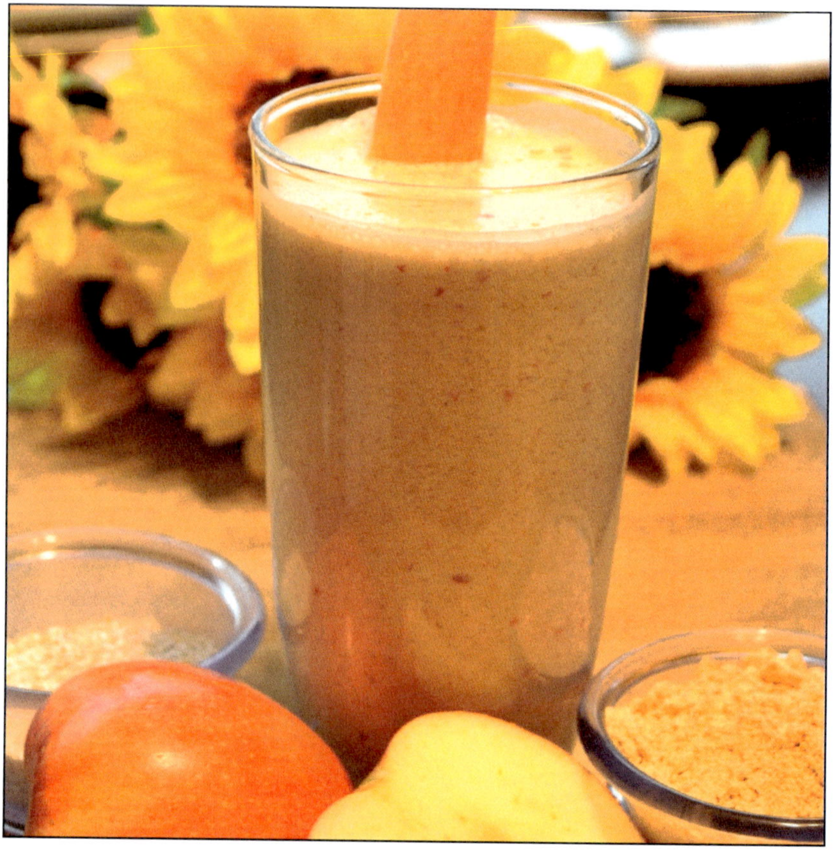

Yes, it is possible to create a healthy peanut butter shake! It's the smoothie equivalent of apple slices with PB, with the antioxidant bonus from the moringa powder. Kids will love this tasty treat.

Ingredients

- 2 celery stalks
- 1 red apple, seeded & quartered
- 2 tablespoons natural peanut butter or peanut butter substitute
- 1 cup unsweetened almond milk
- 1 tbsp. moringa powder
- 1 teaspoon vanilla extract
- ¾ cup ice cubes

Your Notes

47. Basil Grape Elixir

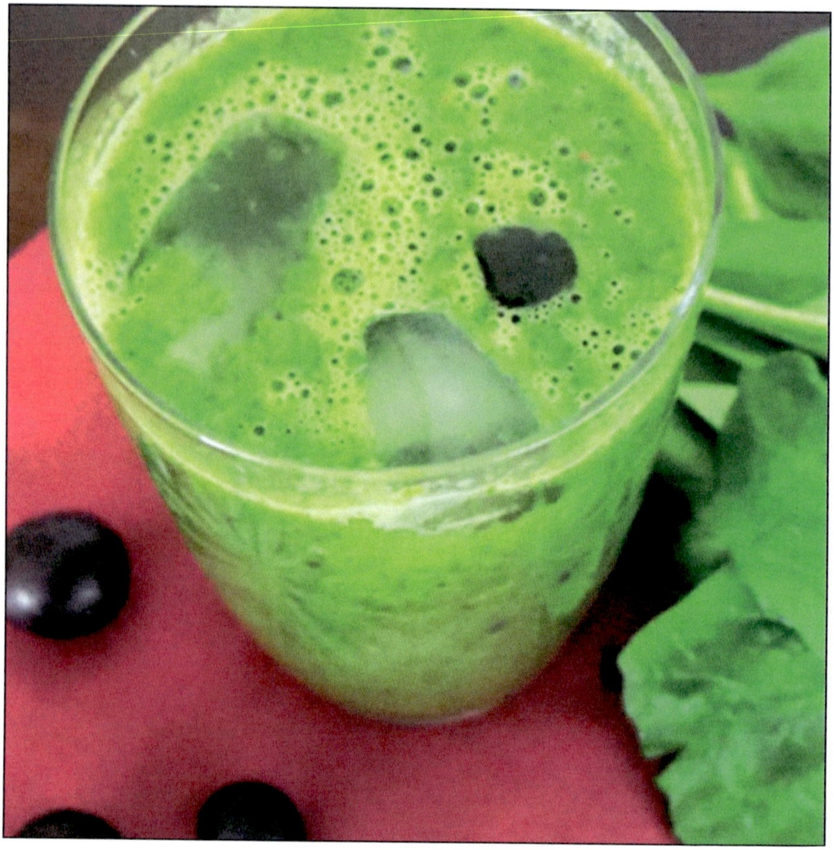

This green smoothie elixir is perfect for preventing oxidative stress and reducing inflammation. The lemon basil combo works just as well in your drink as it does in your favorite pesto.

Ingredients

- 5 leaves fresh basil
- 3 cups spinach
- 1 cup red grapes
- 2 celery sticks
- ½ lemon, peeled and seeded
- 1 cup water

Your Notes

48. Lucuma Blackberry Pudding

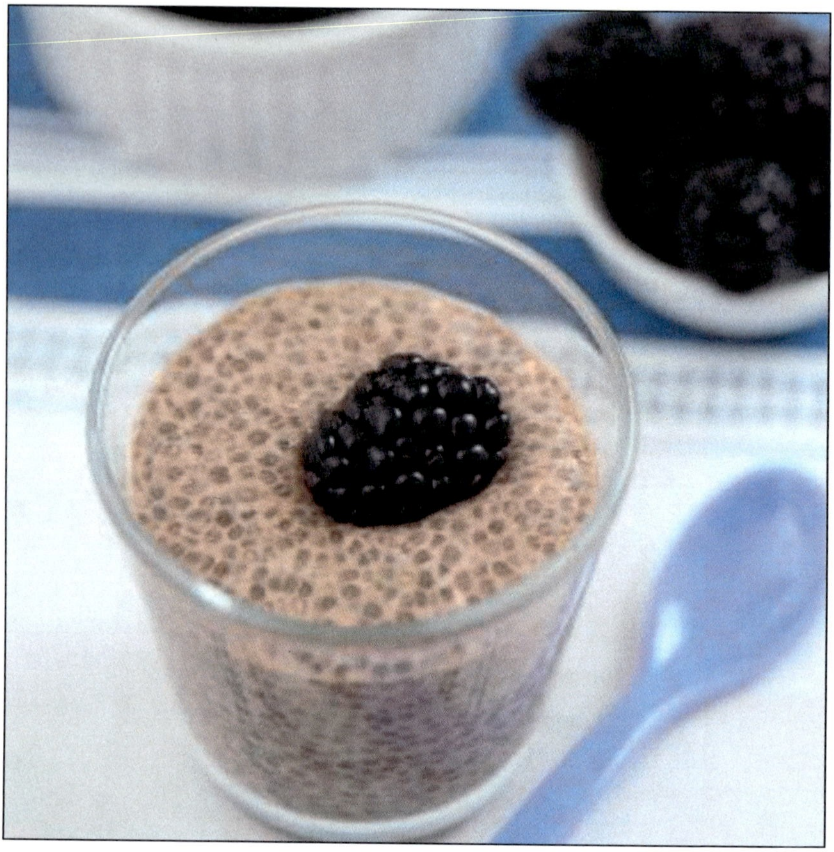

This pudding can be blended and eaten as a smoothie, or it can be prepared ahead of time and allowed to reach more of a pudding consistency as the chia seeds hydrate and swell.

Lucuma powder comes from the lucuma fruit, native to Peru, Ecuador, and Chile. In addition to serving as a natural sweetener, it provides 14 essential trace elements. If you are diabetic, lucuma will not raise blood sugar levels. Keep it in your pantry for sweetening beverages, pastries, etc.

Ingredients

- 1/4 cup chia seeds
- 1 cup coconut milk
- 1/2 tbsp. lucuma powder
- 1/2 tbsp. maca powder
- top with blackberries

Your Notes

49. Hazelnut Ginger Smoothie

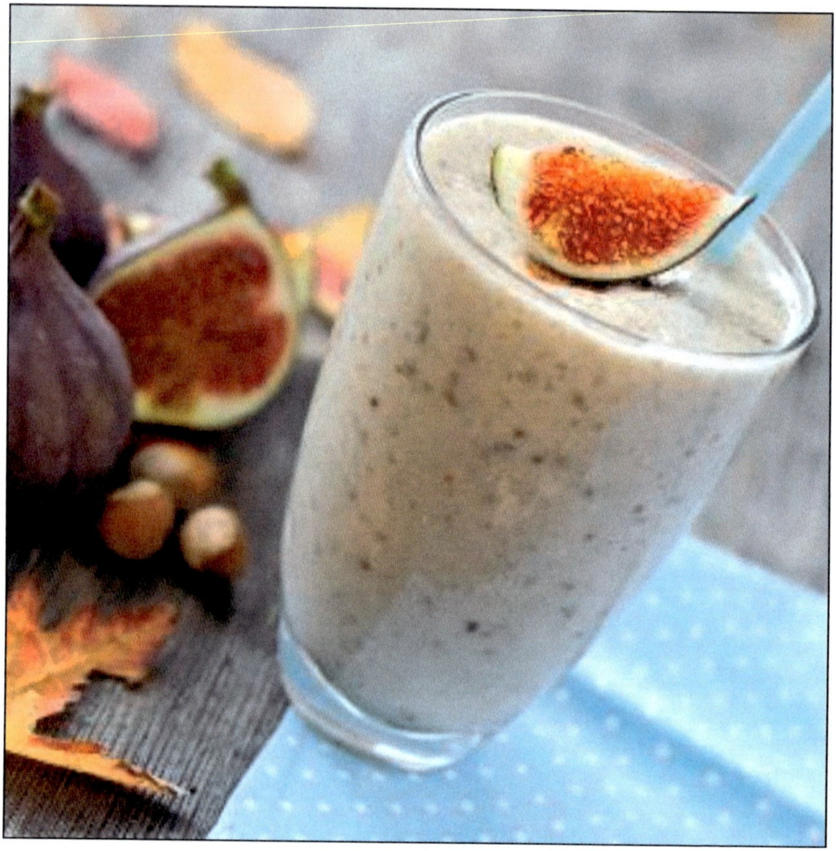

Don't be afraid to really embrace healthy fats in your smoothies. When combined with clean proteins and complex carbohydrates, that's how you turn a smoothie into a meal. This Hazelnut Ginger Smoothie tastes like a crisp fall morning. If you drink coffee, it goes well with a shot of espresso or some cold brew.

Ingredients

- 1 cup unsweetened rice milk
- 1 cup cauliflower florets
- 2 figs
- Juice of ½ lemon
- 1/2 cup ice
- 1 tbsp. fresh ginger
- 1 tbsp. maca powder
- 6-8 hazelnuts

Your Notes

50. Coconut Chia Pudding

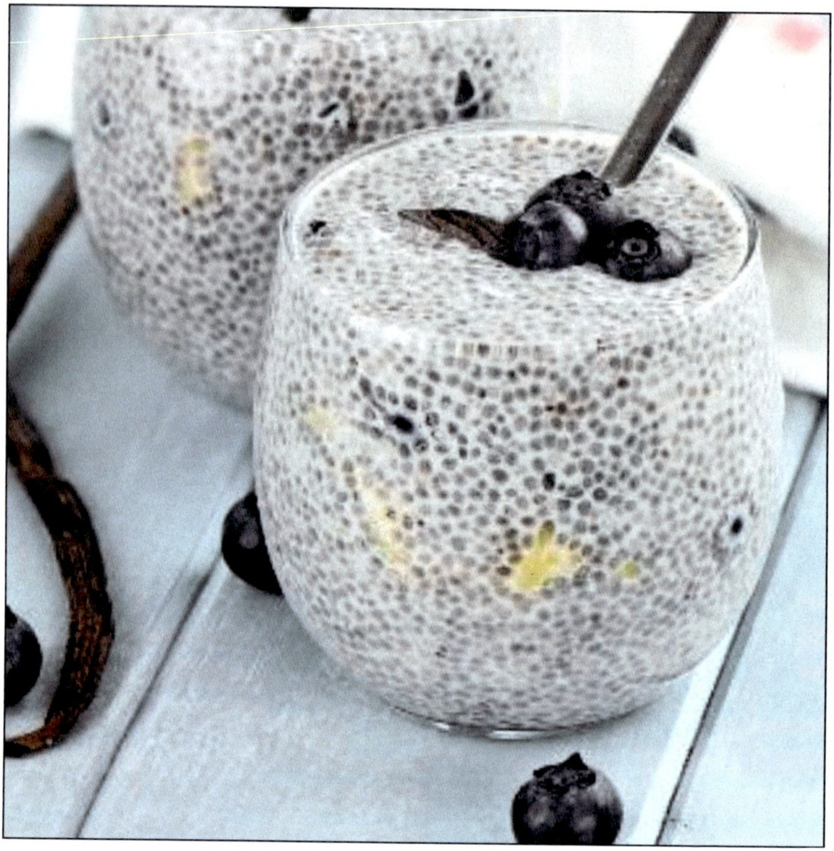

Those who are new to chia puddings will love how simple this is to make. Combine all ingredients except the blueberries, and give the pudding about 10 minutes to thicken. The chia seeds are loaded with omega-3 fatty acids, which help to raise “good” cholesterol levels.

Ingredients

- 1/4 cup chia seeds
- 1 cup coconut milk
- 1 tsp. vanilla extract
- Pinch nutmeg
- Top with blueberries

Your Notes

About the Author

Dr. Duc Vuong helps people break free from unwanted patterns and limiting beliefs so that they can start over and be more. Although he began his career as an internationally renowned bariatric surgeon, who is the world's leading expert in education for the bariatric patient, his methodologies work for any person in any area of life.

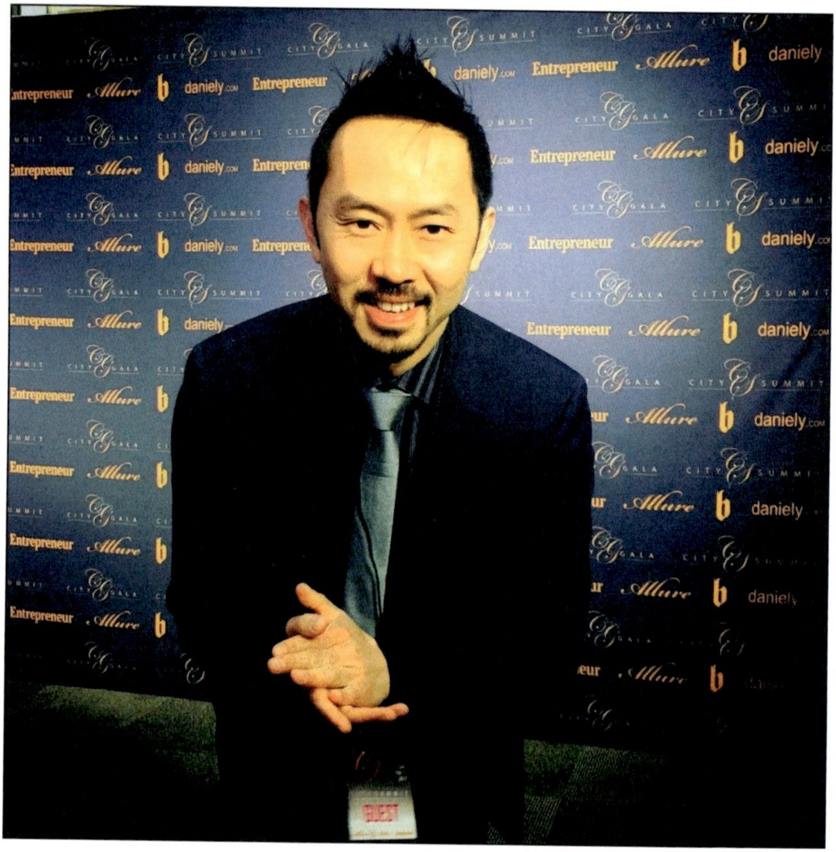

Trained in Western medicine, he blends traditional Eastern teachings with the latest in science and technology. Dr. Vuong was featured in TLC's hit show, 900 Pound Man: Race Against

Time, and is currently working on his own weekly television show. He is the author of multiple Amazon best selling books.

Meet Dr. V in person at one of his LIVE EVENTS:

www.drvtours.com

Visit Dr. Duc Vuong on social media:

www.Facebook.com/doctorvuong

www.youtube.com/user/DoctorVuong

on Instagram @DrDucVuong

www.DucVuong.com

Other Books by Dr. Duc Vuong

(available on Amazon.com)

Ultimate Gastric Sleeve Success: A Practical Patient Guide

Eating Healthy on a Budget

Eating Healthy For Kids

Love is Fishy: 31 Delicious Fish Recipes Told Through a Love Story

Meditate to Lose Weight: A Guide For A Slimmer Healthier You

Healthy Green Smoothies: 50 Easy Recipes That Will Change Your Life

Big-Ass Salads: 31 Easy Recipes For Your Healthy Month

Weight Loss Surgery Success: Dr. V's A-Z Steps For Losing Weight And Gaining Enlightenment

Lap-Band Rescue: Revisit. Rethink. Revise.

Top 30 Exercise Myths

Duc It Up!: 366 Tips To Improve Your Life